Your
PENIS

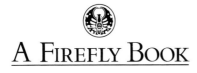

A FIREFLY BOOK

Published by Firefly Books Ltd. 2021
First published in French by Mango, Paris, France — 2020
© Mango, Paris, 2020

First printing

Library of Congress Control Number: 2020950238

Library and Archives Canada Cataloguing in Publication
Title: Your penis : everything you need to know about your friend! / Dr. Michel Lenois ;
    illustrations, Lisa Laubreaux ; translation, Adriana Paradiso.
Other titles: Zizi. English
Names: Lenois, Michel, author. | Laubreaux, Lisa, illustrator. | Paradiso, Adriana, translator.
Description: Translation of: Le zizi.
Identifiers: Canadiana 20200391224 | ISBN 9780228103226 (softcover)
Subjects: LCSH: Penis—Popular works. | LCSH: Generative organs, Male—Popular works. |
LCSH: Human
    reproduction—Popular works.
Classification: LCC QP253 .L4613 2021 | DDC 612.6/16—dc23

Published in Canada by
Firefly Books Ltd.
50 Staples Avenue, Unit 1
Richmond Hill, Ontario
L4B 0A7

Published in the United States by
Firefly Books (U.S.) Inc.
P.O. Box 1338, Ellicott Station
Buffalo, New York
14205

Translation: Adriana Paradiso
Layout: Catherine Le Troquier
Slang compiled by Mark Haebner

Printed in Canada

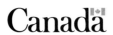

We acknowledge the financial support of the Government of Canada.

Your PENIS

Everything You Need to Know About Your Friend!

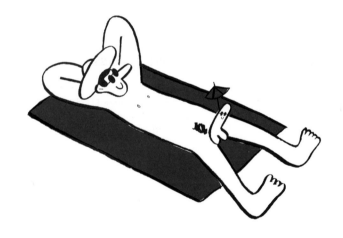

Dr. Michel Lenois

Illustrations : Lisa Laubreaux

FIREFLY BOOKS

CONTENTS

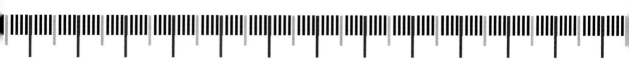

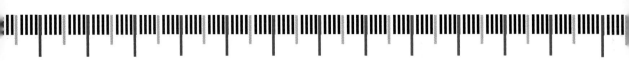

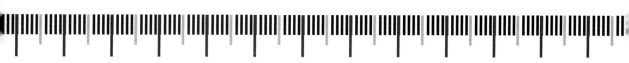

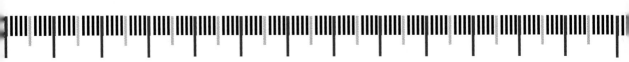

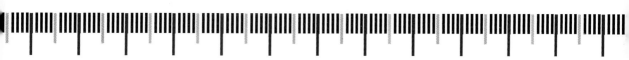

Introduction

Maybe you're very aware of it, or maybe you only think about it every once in a while. We often hear about it, especially in terms of its size. The "it" being referred to is, of course, the penis.

The aim of this book is to provide a comprehensive overview of the penis by discussing its anatomy but also the mechanism of an erection, which engages hydraulic and biochemical processes. We also broach the thorny issue of size and the different disorders that can alter how the penis functions.

But what is a normal penis? Are there different types? And what about famous penises like those of Rasputin or Rocco Siffredi? Did you know a penis can be a shower or a grower? Or that a donkey's penis is on average 15.75 inches (40 cm) long when erect, while an octopus's is detachable? Have you ever heard of techniques to modify a penis, such as the bite from a particular snake or the insertion of pieces of a toothbrush underneath the skin?

With a medically sound but humorous approach, I hope to inform and entertain you and, above all, convince you of the penis's discreet charm.

Anatomy

To understand the penis's composition, we are going to slice it (not literally!) crosswise (see figure 1). We will then cut it lengthwise (see figure 2). It should be noted that the drawings are accurate but very simplified. Only the elements directly relating to our topic will be shown, which explains the absence of various nearby organs, even though some of them are part of the reproductive or urinary systems.

Lateral Cross Section of the Penis

The skin covering the penis can sometimes have small, whitish bumps that are evenly distributed on its surface. They are especially noticeable during an erection. Adolescents and young men often needlessly worry about them. They are called Fordyce spots and correspond to sebaceous glands located just under the skin. Their growth is stimulated by male hormones, hence their appearance around puberty. Fordyce spots are not pathological; they are completely harmless, present in approximately half of young men, and do not require treatment. They often disappear with age. In girls, these same spots are frequently found on the labia minora.

The deep dorsal vein (1) and the two corpora cavernosa (5) are found on the dorsal (top) side of the penis, under the skin. The root of the corpora cavernosa extends into the body, well beyond the penis, under the perineum. Each corpus cavernosum is roughly the shape of a cylinder. They are arranged side by side, and both can fill with blood, allowing them to function together during an erection.

Arteries, aptly called the cavernous arteries (4), run lengthwise through each corpus cavernosum and supply them with blood. The structure of the corpora cavernosa is a series of trabeculae (small bundles of fibers that form a framework) that create sinusoidal spaces, giving

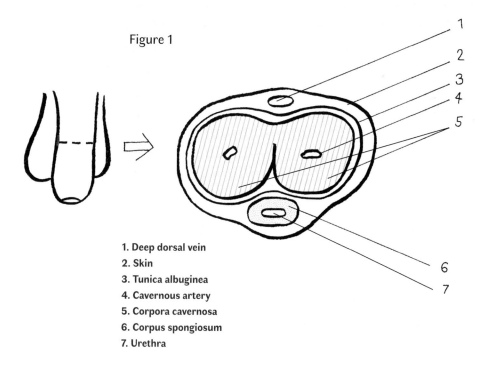

Figure 1

1
2
3
4
5

1. Deep dorsal vein
2. Skin
3. Tunica albuginea
4. Cavernous artery
5. Corpora cavernosa
6. Corpus spongiosum
7. Urethra

6
7

it a spongelike composition. The outside of the corpora cavernosa is covered by a tough, whitish membrane called the tunica albuginea (3).

Once engorged with blood, the corpora cavernosa become rigid, enabling an erection (there is a whole chapter dedicated to erections that details this process; see pages 31–37).

On the ventral (bottom) side of the penis is the corpus spongiosum (6), which also has a roughly cylindrical shape and is enveloped by the tunica albuginea. It contains the urethra (7), which is a tube that expels urine and sperm from the body. During an erection, the corpus spongiosum also swells due to a rush of blood, but it will not become as rigid as the corpora cavernosa. That's a good thing, since the urethra, which is inside it, remains permeable and allows sperm to pass through.

Longitudinal Cross Section of the Penis

This view of the penis also presents the corpus spongiosum (4) and urethra (5), but it also shows the bulge at the end of the corpus spongiosum known as the glans penis (7). The glans is covered by a fold of skin called the foreskin (6).

Figure 2 shows that a fibrous zone called the suspensory ligament (2) connects the corpora cavernosa to the pubic bone (1). This ligament helps support the penis in the proper position (generally upward) during an erection.

Plastic surgeons offer — for a high price and with no guarantee of success — treatments that supposedly elongate the penis by cutting this suspensory ligament. We explore this in detail in the chapter dedicated to various methods proposed for elongating the penis (see pages 61–75).

The length of the penis can vary greatly from one individual to the next and even for the same individual, depending on the circum-

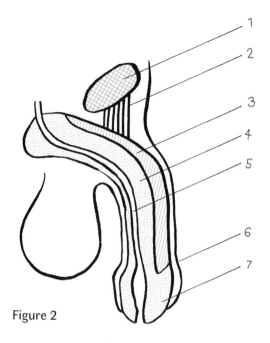

Figure 2

1. Pubic bone
2. Suspensory ligament
3. Corpus cavernosum
4. Corpus spongiosum
5. Urethra
6. Foreskin
7. Glans penis

stances. The penis tends to retract when it is cold and during stressful events, due to the effect of adrenaline, which is a hormone secreted by the body in response to danger. Culturally, penis size holds great importance, and there is a whole chapter dedicated to the topic (see pages 38–60).

The foreskin (6) is a movable fold of skin that covers the glans and helps retain moisture on its surface. The inner side of the foreskin has glands that most likely secrete pheromones (substances that can influence behavior, particularly sexual behavior, through smell). The existence of pheromones has been demonstrated in many animals, but there is no consensus on their existence in humans.

During an erection, the foreskin will slide back, or unfold so to speak. That allows the penis to lengthen. The inner surface of the foreskin also has sensory receptors called Krause's corpuscles, which make it a very sensitive erogenous zone.

The foreskin's open end is sometimes referred to as the preputial ring. In adults, it is typically elastic enough to allow the glans to pass through during an erection. However, the preputial ring can sometimes be too tight to let the glans through. This condition is called phimosis. Phimosis is common in children and does not pose any specific health concerns. Until recently, physicians would recommend that parents regularly pull back the foreskin if their child was experiencing phimosis, using a bit of force if necessary. Today, most medical professionals agree it's best to leave things as they are. Later, when a boy experiences his first erections during puberty, phimosis usually disappears on its own, aided by the nightly routine of manual manipulation at that age.

Another curiosity relating to the foreskin is penile adhesions. These result from the inner foreskin adhering to the base of the glans. They are common in children and should be examined by a physician. In the past, physicians tended to intervene a bit brutally and separate these adhesions by lifting them with a metal probe. However, the only complication associated with these adhesions is their tendency to retain smegma (a foul-smelling, whitish discharge produced by sebaceous glands found along the rim of the glans). As with phimosis, erections will naturally release these adhesions during puberty.

Circumcision is a surgical procedure to remove the foreskin. It is done for religious as well as hygienic reasons. Because of its importance in terms of religion, culture and health, an entire chapter has been dedicated to the topic (see pages 156–166).

The Glans Penis

At right is the anatomy of the glans penis (2), commonly known as the head or tip of the penis. We can see the opening of the urethra,

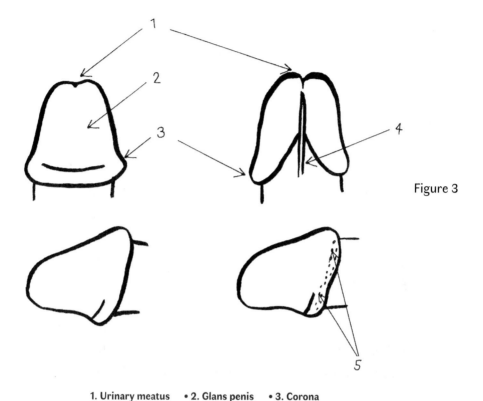

Figure 3

1. Urinary meatus • 2. Glans penis • 3. Corona
• 4. Frenulum • 5.Excrescences

called the urinary meatus (1), as well as the rim located at the base of the glans, called the corona (3). Under this rim is the balanopreputial fold.

Men sometimes have excrescences (5), which are small bumps on the corona of the glans and evenly spaced around its entire periphery. These are gland openings typically found in this area that have become enlarged due to the effects of male hormones. Most physicians have been visited by men who are worried about these small growths on their genitals. It is not a disease, but rather an anatomical curiosity called pearly penile papules, and they do not require any treatment.

Pearly penile papules are found mainly in young men, generally from puberty and into their 30s who have high levels of male hormones. These papules often gradually disappear with age and are generally not found in older men.

The frenulum (4) is a membranous fold on the top side of the glans penis. It begins at the urinary meatus. In some males, the frenulum is abnormally short and can tear during sexual intercourse. We discuss this situation in a chapter dedicated to health problems relating to the penis (see pages 107–111). Similar to the inside of the foreskin, the frenulum has numerous microscopic formations, like the previously mentioned Krause's corpuscles, which are sensory receptors linked to pleasure.

Hey, are we cousins?

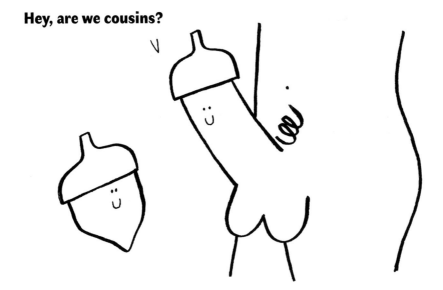

Transection of the Penis

Figure 4 shows a cross section of the various elements of the penis's anatomy that we have just reviewed, providing a better perspective of their arrangement in the human body.

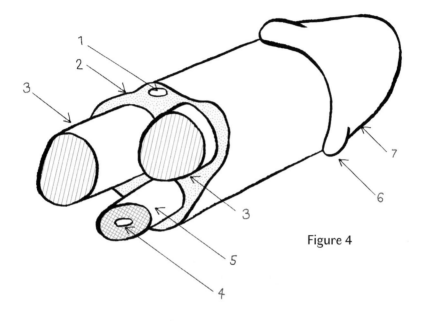

Figure 4

1. Dorsal vein   2. Skin   3. Corpus cavernosum   4. Urethra
5. Corpus spongiosum   6. Corona   7. Glans penis

What About the Color?

A person's skin color, be it lighter or darker, is caused by melanin, which is a pigment produced by cells in the epidermis called melanocytes. Compared to white people, the amount of melanin is about ten times greater in people of African ancestry and five to six times greater in people of Asian ancestry. However, an individual's skin color can change over time.

Melanin also protects people from ultraviolet rays, and an increase in its production is what creates a tan. In the absence of melanin, the skin remains white, as is the case with albinism. The absence of melanin, and the protection it offers from the ultraviolet rays, leads people with albinism to be extremely sensitive to the sun's rays and to have higher rates of skin cancers.

In childhood, the reproductive organs, and particularly the penis, are the same color as the rest of the body. During puberty, these areas get progressively darker. In males, this is visible in the scrotum and penis, and in females in the labia majora. In both sexes, the areolas of the breasts also become darker. This change is caused by sex hormones: testosterone in males and estrogen in females.

In people with albinism, the lack of melanin leads to a very white skin color, but there are also conditions that cause localized skin discolorations, such as vitiligo. This condition causes small or large areas of skin to discolor due to a loss of melanocytes. Vitiligo can affect any part of the body, but it most commonly affects the hands, elbows, knees and reproductive organs of both sexes, particularly the penis. A certain famous African-American pop star who has now passed may therefore have had a white colored penis. Vitiligo is a partly genetic condition, and its progression is linked to the affected person's physical state. Stress tends to cause flare-ups.

Can the Penis Tan?

The penis's skin does, of course, contain melanocytes. If it is exposed to sunlight, these melanocytes secrete a large quantity of melanin, which is the body's defense mechanism against ultraviolet rays. The exposed area will get progressively darker, so it is quite possible to tan your penis! Melanocytes are also found in the glans, and this area can also tan, but it is very delicate, and exposure to the sun will quickly cause a very painful sunburn.

Medical Imaging of the Penis

On a standard X-ray, the penis appears as a shadow, which has inspired orthopedic surgeons to come up with the concept of the "John Thomas sign." John Thomas is slang for the penis, and the John Thomas sign is associated with femoral neck fractures and can be positive or negative. The John Thomas sign is said to be positive when the penis's shadow points toward the same side as the fracture; it is said to be negative when the shadow points toward the opposite side to the fracture. This is all in good fun, of course, as the John Thomas sign has no diagnostic value.

On a more serious note, the inside of a penis can be viewed via ultrasound, but an MRI is the technique of choice for getting detailed images. They allow us to perform various diagnostics, such as assessing traumatic damage to the organ and perform other diagnoses.

What Are Animal Penises Like?

"The kangaroo has a double penis – one for week days and one for holidays."
— Henry Miller, *Tropic of Cancer*

Split in two, extraordinarily large, strangely shaped, capable of producing sounds, equipped with a locking function or a bone, able to function autonomously and detach from its owner to fertilize the female — animal penises are often very different from humans' members. Let's take a closer look at some examples.

Hung like a Donkey!

This flattering expression alludes to this animal's very respectable penis length. Zoologists have not shied away, ruler in hand, from measuring the size of a donkey's erect penis, some of which can be almost 16 inches (40 cm) long. Moreover, some particularly resourceful donkeys take advantage of their penis's length to perform auto-fellatio!

In China, donkey penis is considered by some to be an aphrodisiac and is eaten for that purpose. It is prepared in various ways and, of course, presented on a platter in its entirety. This dish has contributed to the animal's dwindling numbers in both China and Africa. In the past few years, millions of South African donkeys have been killed by animal traffickers and their penises sent to China.

Paper Nautilus

This close relative of the octopus has an extraordinary penis, called a hectocotylus. It is actually one of the animal's arms, which contains sperm and can detach from its body. Once separated, the hectocotylus swims to the female, which captures it and uses it to fertilize her eggs. Nature knows best though: the hectocotylus grows back for the next mating season.

Blue Whales

A blue whale's penis often reaches 10 feet (3 m) in length, while its body is generally 100 feet (30 m) long. Cetaceans (a broad group of mammals that includes dolphins and whales) once walked on land. They therefore had a pelvic bone. While they have been underwater creatures for a very long time, they still retain this pelvic bone. Scientists once believed it was vestigial (meaning it was simply a leftover from the past), but some are proposing that it still serves a purpose. They theorize Mr. Whale can steer his penis and perhaps even provide pleasure to his partner. There is a potential advantage here: Females may be more likely to reproduce with a male with whom they enjoy mating.

With everything being proportional, Mr. Whale ejaculates 5 gallons (20 l) of sperm every time he has sex, compared to 0.5 to 1 teaspoons (2–5 ml) for humans, This is not really not surprising, since each of his testicles weighs some 130 pounds (60 kg), compared to 0.75 ounces (20 g) for humans.

Homebody Hermit Crabs

If you've spent time at the beach, you may well have encountered hermit crabs. These small shell-less crustaceans have found a way to protect their soft, defenseless bodies by squatting in empty shells. Thus protected, they hold little interest as a food source, have low levels of predation and are abundant in the pools of water left behind by the tide. There are also varieties of land hermit crabs in many hot climates, and these animals are very useful to the environment: They clean beaches by feeding on

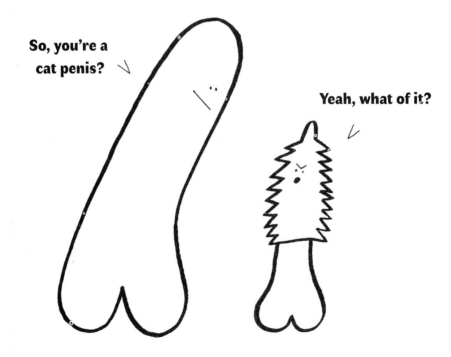

trash, plant debris and the carcasses of marine animals washed up on shore. One species of land hermit crab, called *Coenobita perlatus*, deserves a mention in this chapter. To reproduce, hermit crabs need to leave their shell and, once naked, become easy prey. The male *Coenobita perlatus* has solved this problem by disproportionately extending his penis, which allows him to fertilize the female while remaining safe in his shell.

Cats

Female cats have the physiological distinction of only ovulating once sex is complete. Tomcats, meanwhile, have a penis with many small, rearward-facing spikes. Penile spines (the scientific term) stimulate their partner's vaginal wall and thus trigger ovulation. What's more, when the penis is in place, it is solidly held in by the erected penile spines, and they cannot be retracted until after ejaculation.

Knotty Dogs

The visible, red part of a dog's erected penis consists only of the glans penis. A dog's glans is composed of the elongated front section and a bulbous back section called the bulbus glandis, which is responsible for a knotting phenomenon. Once the canine's penis has entered the vagina, the bulbus glandis swells and prevents it from coming out until ejaculation has occurred. In addition, the dogs, which started in the doggy-style position, will rotate a half turn and end up in a backside-to-backside position.

Like many animals, dogs have a penis bone, called a baculum. It is a floating bone that characteristically is not attached to the rest of the skeleton. The baculum helps make the dog's penis rigid, which is necessary for mating.

Short-Beaked Echidnas

This close relative of the platypus has some truly remarkable features: They are mammals, but the female lays eggs and her milk is pink. Another curiosity: Mrs. Echidna has two vaginas, but Mr. Echidna is even better off — he has a four-headed penis.

African Elephants

An African elephant measures 11.5 feet (3.5 m) at the shoulders, weighs 5.5 to 9 tons (5–8 metric tons), and the male's erect penis measures 6.5 feet (2 m), which is the same length as his trunk!

Two-in-One Snails

Snails are hermaphrodites. They produce both sperm and eggs, but they cannot fertilize themselves, so they need a partner to reproduce. During foreplay, which lasts half a day, the two partners stimulate each other by shooting each other with their "love dart," which are a kind of calcareous dart located on one side of their bodies. Then the two snails mutually fertilize each other by sticking their penis in their partner's genital opening.

Gorillas

The gorilla penis is barely visible in its flaccid state and does not exceed 2 inches (5 cm) when erect. Note that the gorilla also has a baculum. This bone acts as a support for the penis in many other primates, but not in humans, who lost it hundreds of thousands of years ago.

Spotted Hyenas

For a very long time, people who lived around hyenas believed that female hyenas did not exist. This is because their clitoris is so large that it resembles a penis. In spotted hyenas, the similarity is so great that it is utterly impossible to distinguish between males and females. Only an autopsy can reveal the difference between the two sexes. Another unique feature: hyenas give birth through their hypertrophied clitoris.

Female Neotrogla Wear the Pants

Few people know about the *Neotrogla* species. Nevertheless, this small animal is quite extraordinary! It is a small flying insect, about 0.1 inch (3 mm) long, that lives in caves in Brazil. It was only recently discovered in 2010. Its distinction, unique in the animal kingdom, is that the female has a penis, which scientists have named the gynosome. This term combines two Greek words and literally means "female body."

When Neotrogla mate, the female climbs onto her partner and penetrates his body with her gynosome. Spines located on the member ensures a solid anchoring throughout the act, which is particularly long — *Neotrogla* sex lasts two to three days. The scientists who studied this unusual breeding have tried to separate the two partners and only succeeded in tearing the male in two. Once the male *Neotrogla* is impaled, the female collects sperm from within his body as well as many nutrients, which will allow her to carry out the spawning. It should be said that food is rare in the *Neotrogla*'s environment, and these insects feed mainly on the bodies of dead bats.

All truly scientific work has value, although some studies are almost certainly more valuable than others. In 2017, the researchers who studied the *Neotrogla* (two Japanese, a Brazilian and a Swiss) received the Ig Nobel Prize (a parody prize of the real Nobel Prize), which is awarded each year to 10 scientists who have conducted "research that makes people laugh and then think."

Not Many Small Worms for Birds

Most birds have a cloaca, which is a cavity that contains the end of the digestive tract (and carries excrement), the bladder (which expels urine), and the reproductive organs. In most birds, fertilization takes place by the touching of cloacae: As the male holds his cloaca against the female's cloaca, sperm eventually find its way.

Ostriches, geese, swans and ducks are some of the rare birds with a penis. The penis of the Argentine lake duck, which looks like a corkscrew, is quite large, and ornithologists have found some that have reached the respectable length of 16.5 inches (42 cm) once outside of the body.

Winking Seven-armed Octopuses

Haliphron atlanticus is an octopus whose arm span can measure more than 6.5 feet (2 m) long. It appears to have only seven arms. However, like the etymology of its name indicates, any good octopod must have eight. In reality, one of its arms is located in a pocket near its right eye. It is called a hectocotylus and is the equivalent to a penis. During mating, this appendage deposits sperm into the female's genital opening. As with the *Paper nautilus*, its hectocotylus detaches itself from the male and is kept by the female inside her body.

The Serenade of the Water Bug

We sometimes see insects such as water bugs moving quickly along the top of a pond and other body of water. One such insect, called *Micronecta scholtzi*, is tiny, measuring only 0.08 inches (2 mm) long, but it appears in the *Guinness World Records* book as the loudest animal in the world relative to its size. To attract females, the male *M. scholtzi* rubs its penis against its abdomen. This technique is effective, as noted by entomologists who measured the intensity of this serenade to be more than 99 dB.

The Bedbug and Its Spicule

Bedbugs (*Cimex lectularius*) are tiny insects that can infest soft materials, such bedding and mattresses, hence their common name. With the introduction of DDT and other powerful insecticides, bedbugs had practically disappeared in many countries by the mid-20th century. After DDT was banned due to its horrific effects on the environment, these troublesome insects came back with a bang. Bedbugs are commonly compared to a reddish-brown lentil measuring 0.2 to 0.3 inches (5–8 mm) in diameter. This pest feeds exclusively on blood, often from unsuspecting people as they sleep. Nature knows best, so to speak, because once the victim has been bitten, the bedbug injects them with an anesthetic and anticoagulant. Therefore, the bite is painless, and no clot interrupts its bloody meal.

In humans, their bite leads to small red spots that are often arranged in a line or a cluster. Extra-sensitive people can sometimes experience an allergic reaction that causes intense itchiness.

Let's get back to the bedbug itself. The male has a very sharp penis (the scientific term is spicule), which he uses to puncture the female's body during mating to deposit his sperm. Entomologists call this process traumatic insemination. Quite frequently, bedbugs get the wrong target and couple up with other males. The injected sperm is not all lost, though — it survives in the receiving male and will be injected with his own sperm when he later mates with a female.

Snakes and Lizards

Snakes and lizards have the distinction of having two close-set penises. They retract their penis into their body, and it comes out, erect, only during reproduction. The penises of most snakes and lizards have scales and spikes, sometimes even hooks. Herpetologists, those who specialize in the study of reptiles, have noted an unexpected phenomenon involving the penis among some snakes: Once the scaly, spiky or hooked penis is inside the female's cloaca, it is firmly secured, and if the couple is disturbed mid-action, Mrs. Snake will drag her partner out of the way to finish what they started.

The Icelandic Phallological Museum

The world of animal penises is immense and presents so many varieties that it is not possible to describe all of them in this chapter. If this subject interests you, you would certainly enjoy the unique and entertaining Icelandic Phallological Museum.

Here you will see 282 penis specimens from 93 animal species, from a humble hamster penis to a whopper of a whale penis. Since 2011, the human species is represented by a (postmortem!) donation from Pall Arason.

Erections

"The penis — if you think about it — is the most enterprising engineering feat imaginable — a cantilevered structure, hydraulics, propulsion, pistons, compression, inflation, heat sensitive — practically every engineering characteristic — towers, draw-bridges, rocket-ships — no man-made engineering structure to match it."
— Peter Greenaway

There is something magical about an erection. Here's an organ that doesn't look like much when resting, but it doubles in size, if not more, while becoming rigid in response to a caress, a thought, the sight of a someone desirable — and even when dreaming. Most men benefit from their erections without having the slightest clue of the inner workings, kind of like a driver who uses their car every day without knowing what's under the hood or what kind of motor makes it go. Luckily, some people are more curious than others and want to know how things work. Here are a few explanations for those who want to look under the hood.

A Bit of Hydraulics

The dictionary gives the following definition for the term hydraulic: "operated, moved or effected by means of water."

In the case of the penis we're dealing with blood rather that water, which is what allows the penis to become rigid. The penises of most animals become rigid via blood, while birds have lymph-powered penises.

First, let's quickly review some anatomy. Let's imagine a simplified cross section of the penis in a flaccid state (a medical term that means "not swollen by blood"). As illustrated on page 13, we would find:

- the two corpora cavernosa;
- the two cavernous arteries, one at the center of each corpus cavernosum;
- the superficial dorsal vein, commonly referred to as the big blue vein, on top;
- the circumflex veins on each side;
- the corpus spongiosum on the bottom, which contains the urethra. The corpus spongiosum does not directly contribute to the penis's rigidity; it swells with blood, but it does not become as rigid as the corpora cavernosa. This state allows sperm to pass during ejaculation.

The arrangement we just reviewed is what enables an erection, which occurs as follows:

- Desire, sparked by sensory stimulation, starts in the largest sexual organ we possess: the brain.
- Nerve impulses travel to the spinal cord and then to the pelvic splanchnic nerves.
- In the penis, this desire-turned-nerve-impulse releases nitric oxide (NO), which is a powerful vasodilator.
- NO triggers the cavernous arteries to dilate, an influx of blood fills the corpora cavernosa and the penis starts to swell.

- However, that is not enough to achieve rigidity. A second mechanism intervenes: The corpora cavernosa swell and push the circumflex veins against the outer margins of the penis. The corpora cavernosa then become taut due to the continuous influx of blood that cannot drain, and the penis becomes truly stiff.
- Once ejaculation has occurred, an enzyme intervenes, phosphodiesterase type 5 (called PDE5), and the penis returns to a flaccid state.

Luckily, it's all automatic!

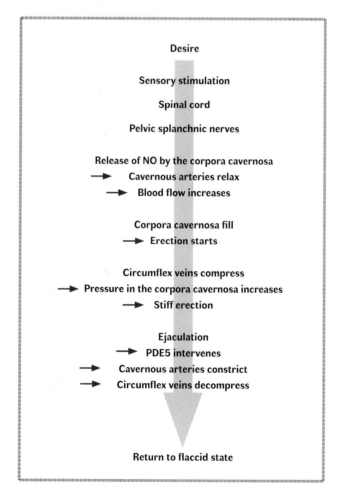

Desire

Sensory stimulation

Spinal cord

Pelvic splanchnic nerves

Release of NO by the corpora cavernosa
→ **Cavernous arteries relax**
→ **Blood flow increases**

Corpora cavernosa fill
→ **Erection starts**

Circumflex veins compress
→ **Pressure in the corpora cavernosa increases**
→ **Stiff erection**

Ejaculation
→ **PDE5 intervenes**
→ **Cavernous arteries constrict**
→ **Circumflex veins decompress**

Return to flaccid state

Knowing about this erectile mechanism will help you better understand why the penis sometimes breaks down and how to fix it.

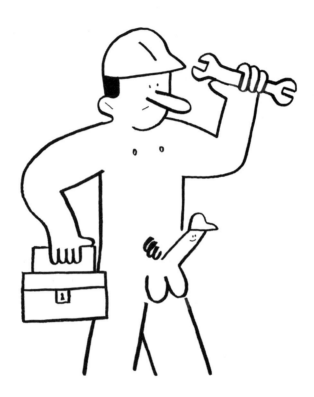

A Bit of Biochemistry

The penis's hydraulic mechanism is supported by a whole sequence of biochemical actions. This chain reaction is helpful to know, as it explains how a drug like Viagra works. Here is the process:

- The NO released in the corpora cavernosa activates an enzyme, called guanylate cyclase, which transforms guanosine triphosphate (GTP) into cyclic guanosine monophosphate (cGMP).
- cGMP triggers vasodilation (widening of the blood vessels), filling the corpora cavernosa with blood, hence causing an erection.
- After ejaculation, another enzyme, called phosphodiesterase type 5 (PDE5), transforms cGMP into GMP, and the erection ends. PDE5 inhibitors facilitate the erection by intervening at this time. In the chapter dedicated to erection problems (see pages 114–121), we will look in detail at drugs like Viagra, Cialis and others.

Shower or Grower

A distinction is made between a shower, a penis that is not much bigger in an erect state than in a flaccid state, and a grower, which significantly increases in size during erection. Conventionally, a penis is called a shower when the length when erect/length at rest ratio is equal to or less than 1.9. If the ratio is greater than that value, it's a grower.

Example of a shower:
- length at rest = 3.5 inches (8.89 cm)
- length when erect = 6 inches (15.24 cm)
- ratio = 1.71

Example of a grower:
- length at rest = 2 inches (5.08 cm)
- length when erect = 6.5 inches (16.51 cm)
- ratio = 3.25

The Refractory Period

Once a male has ejaculated, he cannot just quickly get another erection; he must wait for a period of time, which greatly depends on his age. A young man may be able to have another erection after 15 to 20 minutes, while an older man may have to wait an hour or more. A man in his 60s, meanwhile, may sometimes have to wait a full day. The time between erections is called the refractory period. It is caused by certain hormones, particularly endorphins and oxytocin, which are released during orgasm. It is not possible to shorten the refractory period through medications or other means. This period not only helps cool the jets of eager performers, the hormones involved also facilitate pleasurable post-sex relaxation and encourages bonding and tenderness between partners. We aren't animals! Well, not always anyway.

Nocturnal Erections

Rapid eye movement (REM) sleep, so called because the sleeper rapidly moves their eyes, is the phase of sleep during which we dream. For males, REM sleep is also when nocturnal erections occur. I write "males" and not just "men" because these nocturnal erections also occur in children and the elderly (if they are still in good health). They occur three to five times in a night and generally last 15 to 30 minutes. Researchers who woke up sleepers with an erection and questioned them found that the sleepers were for the most part not having erotic dreams. Desire and nocturnal erections do not seem to be connected.

If one ascribes to the view that nature does nothing in vain (in the sense of uselessness), then these erections must have a function. The most probable explanation is that they help provide oxygen to the penis and keep it in good working order.

Postmortem Erections

Death by hanging often causes an erection, and sometimes even a final ejaculation. In the Middle Ages, the condemned were hanged naked, and their erection was visible to all the spectators. At the time, people believed that the mandrake, a plant widely used by healers to make different concoctions, grew from the earth fertilized by that final sperm.

The physiological explanation of this erection is not clear and there is no consensus about why it occurs. Some attribute it to cerebral damage caused by the rope, others attribute it to a rush of blood toward the body's lower half, and others still to a lack of oxygen.

A somewhat macabre and very dangerous sex game referred to as erotic asphyxiation involves beginning to hang oneself to elicit an erection. From time to time, media report deaths resulting from such acts. Some 20 years ago, American health authorities estimated several hundred deaths per year were caused by pseudo-hangings for erotic purposes that went wrong.

Big Penis?
Small Penis?

**"Don't judge a peppercorn by its size.
Taste it, and you will feel its bite."
Arab proverb**

For the ancient Greeks, a small penis seems to have been the ideal of masculine beauty, as their statues that have survived are endowed with modestly sized penises. The Romans adopted the same model. For them, a large penis was completely vulgar. Today, the Indigenous Tucano people of Colombia reserve the highest social duties for men whose penis "does not exceed the size of a hummingbird."

However, the Tucano people are a modern exception, since big penises are now valued and being called a "needle dick" is not well received. But what size of penis is considered small? What is a "normal" size? We wear clothes in our daily lives, so unless you are a naturalist or a part of certain medical professions, it is difficult to get a sense of a "normal" penis size and assess your own. Worse, the omnipresence of pornography on the Internet gives many people a completely exaggerated idea of penis size. It shows porn stars with oversized members, not Mr. Average with an ordinary, "normal" penis.

Studies have been done by scientists, doctors and anthropologists, who have spent time measuring penises and creating graphs to find averages. Here are some of their findings.

First, How Do You Measure a Penis?

Penis length is measured from the pubis to the tip of the glans, and the circumference is measured at the midpoint. There is one problem with using a ruler to measure a penis: The scale on most rulers does not begin right at the edge but at around a quarter of an inch from the edge; this should be taken into account. The most practical way to measure a penis's circumference is to use a tape measure, but a ruler should allow you to make an initial assessment.

The conditions during which the measurements are taken also matter. All men know that the penis retracts and gets soft when it's cold. It also retracts when affected by adrenaline, when a man experiences fear or apprehension. It is therefore necessary to measure a penis in a warm enough place and on a totally relaxed individual.

Some studies are biased, and their results are overstated, simply because the subjects themselves took their own measurements. With no one watching, it is easy and tempting to give oneself an extra half inch or so, boosting the ego because having a big penis is valued.

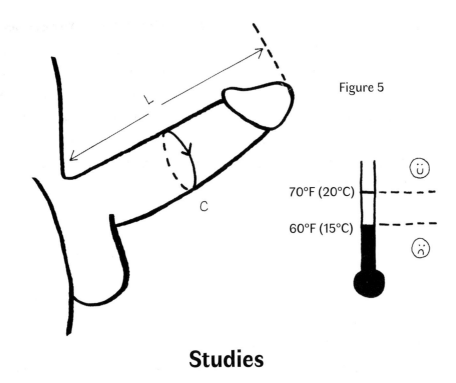

Figure 5

70°F (20°C)

60°F (15°C)

Studies

Khérumian and Juster: Two Trailblazers

In 1948, a researcher by the name of B. R. Khérumian published a study in a French journal that examined the penis lengths of men from Central Europe. This study was probably read by only a few scholars, which is a shame because it is a very interesting document. I was able to locate it it, and here is a translation from the French that indicates how it starts:

> During an anthropological examination of Axis prisoners of war, carried out in 1946–1947, we conducted, among various other observations, the measurement of penis length. Although numerically small, the results that we present could be of interest, given the rarity of statistical documents on this subject matter.

40

We examined 213 men, including 1 Lithuanian, 1 Dane, 1 Yugoslavian, 2 Czechs and 208 Germans (Prussians, Bavarians, Württembergers, Saarlanders, Sudetens, Ripuarians, Hamburgers, Pomeranians, etc.). All our subjects were healthy and normal men, without any notable congenital defects, and all were young or middle aged (20 to 48 years old) and, as a result, without any senile involution. Anthropologically, they made up a heterogenous group, the size varying for example between 154 and 193 cm [60.6–76 inches].

We can imagine these prisoners with their pants pulled down, lining up in front of Khérumian. These men were no doubt a little surprised by what their examiner held in his hand.

In fact, the author specifies how the measurements were taken. He explains how he used a sliding compass and secured the fixed arm at the base of the penis, which he easily identified by the lower edge of the pubic symphysis. He then brought the movable arm closer, without force, to the top of the glans.

But the penis can retract when it's cold. This potential cause of error was not lost on our scientist, who explained in his article that he accounted for other factors that could skew the results, such as low ambient temperatures, which could cause retraction. He confirmed the conditions in which he conducted his study were very favorable, both in terms of the calm demeanor of his subjects and the environment, which was the prisoners' depot infirmary. He specified it was always adequately heated.

Other factors can also skew the results: too low ambient temperature, which can cause retraction [...]. [...] the conditions in which our study was conducted were very favorable, both in terms of the calm demeanor of our subjects and the environment (the prisoners depot infirmary), which was always adequately heated.

Let's take a look at the results: The average among the 213 subjects that Khérumian and his team examined was 88.6 mm (which is about 3.5 inches) and that the degree of variation was significant, with a minimum length of 42 mm (1.7 inches) and a maximum of 128 mm (5 inches).

Further on, the author confirms that there is no correlation between body size and penis length or hair color and penis length. In contrast, he points out that men with blood type O were better endowed than those with blood types B and AB. But what about the thickness of the penises or the diameter? Khérumian surprises us a bit by stating that due to what he termed obvious technical challenges, his team gave up on measuring the circumference of the penis.

What a very curious anthropologist. He has a compass and obviously knows how to use it, but he does not have a simple tape measure? Luckily, he makes up for it a little later in the article, stating his team noted the subjects' testicle size.

The conclusion of this article is full of slightly old-fashioned scientific terminology, as Khérumian notes that resulting from the extremely subtle interplay of heriditary, endocrine and other factors, the individual conformations of a man's sexual organs, whose role is far from being limited to procreation and is often of the determinants of his behavior, warrant the interest of anthropologists and doctors.

Another researcher, Dr. M. Juster, was also interested in the penises of his contemporaries. Two years after Khérumian, he published his observations in a different French journal. Dr. Juster worked on cadavers in the dissection pavilions at the Paris faculty of medicine, and he notes that he studied 129 subjects aged 30 to 90 years old.

His results demonstrate slightly higher values than those of Khérumian, with the shortest specimen at 2.5 inches (65 mm), the longest at 5.5 inches (143 mm) and the average at 4 inches (104 mm).

Like Khérumian, Juster did not find any correlation between body size and penis length. This doctor also extensively studied the glans penis — their owners were not likely offended! — by measuring their diameter, length, length relative to the penis, length covered by the foreskin as well as their shape, making a distinction between cylindrical, conical and cylindroconical glans. Lastly, unlike his predecessor, he had the opportunity to dissect his clients, and he confirmed that he never found a single penis bone.

An Italian Study Published in 2001

This study titled "Penile Length and Circumference: A Study of 3,300 Young Italian Males" was led by Dr. R. Ponchietti. She provides the following averages for penis size: length at rest of 3.5 inches (9 cm), circumference at rest of 4 inches (10 cm) and length during erection of 5 inches (12.5 cm).

A British Study Published in 2015

In this meta-analysis, Dr. David Veale, of King's College London, and his colleagues compiled 20 studies encompassing more than 15,500 men. In all the studies, the penis was measured in accordance with standardized procedure by health professionals, which helped eliminate overly "optimistic" measurements done by the subjects themselves. Here are the results: The average length of a penis at rest is 3.61 inches (9.16 cm). When erect, the average length is 5.17 inches (13.12 cm). The circumference of the penis, on average, goes from 3.61 inches (9.31 cm) at rest to 4.59 inches (11.66 cm) when erect.

A Quick Reminder

Remember that all the studies agree on one thing: There is no correlation between penis size at rest and the size it will become when erect. Some well-sized penises in a flaccid state barely grow, while other more modest penises will double or more in length. These are the so-called showers, which do not change much, and growers, whose size significantly increases once it swells with blood.

What Is a "Normal" Penis Length?

It is difficult to define what is normal for any matter relating to human beings. Merriam-Websters offers these synonyms for the word "normal": average, common, ordinary, standard. This helps us to begin establishing a definition for what normal penis length might be.

For the penis — given that few men have the opportunity to see the penises of others in their everyday life — the comparison is almost always done with what's accessible. Most of the time, the reference will be made by widely circulated porn on the Internet. Since the actors are often chosen for the exceptional length of their member, what serves as the element of comparison is not at all ordinary or common; in other words, normal is quite abnormal. It's no surprise then that 45 percent of men wish they had a bigger, longer penis.

All studies show that the length of the male organ varies greatly from one individual to the next, much more than the size of any other organ. Can you imagine ears or noses whose size difference varies by a factor of three between two people? It is likely that breast sizes among women present the same variation in measurements.

Carl Friedrich Gauss is a famous German mathematician who provided us with, among other things, the bell curve, also known as the Gauss curve. Simply, this curve is used to represent the distribution of a measurement. Here is a drawing that shows its shape:

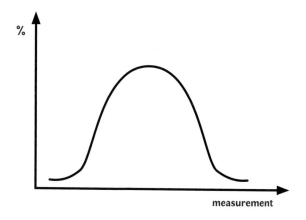

Many human characteristics can be distributed on a bell curve, such as body size, intelligence, physical performances and blood test results. Let's take, for example, IQ, which aims to assess a person's level of intelligence based on test results. These results are distributed as follows:

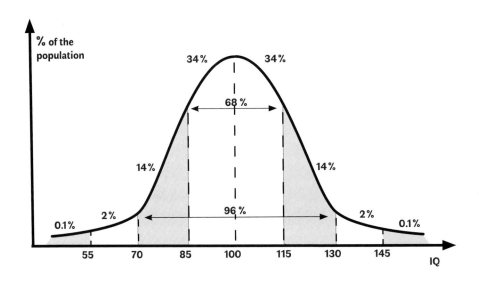

We see that 68 percent of people tested have an IQ ranging between 85 and 115, with a median value of 100. These people are not remarkably intelligent: They are independent and capable of easily holding a conversation and pursuing secondary education.

Meanwhile, 14 percent of people have an IQ ranging between 70 and 85. These people are self-sufficient and may lead a satisfying life, but they are generally not able to pursue studies beyond high school.

A little more than 2 percent of those who were tested have an IQ lower than 70. Those people require assistance in daily life.

On the right of the graph, 14 percent of people have an IQ between 115 and 130. These gifted people can easily pursue postsecondary studies.

A further 2 percent have an IQ above 130: These are geniuses, and there are few of them — only 1 in 50 people.

If we want to talk about what is "normal," we include people who can lead an autonomous and satisfying existence. Therefore, 96 percent of the population could be qualified as "normal."

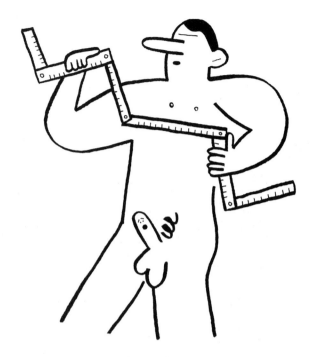

It's the same for penis length. A table in Khérumian's article helps us get a first impression. In total, 75 percent of men studied have a penis measuring between 70 and 99 mm (about 2.75 to 4 inches):

Up to 49	0.93%
50 to 59	0.46%
60 to 69	4.60%
70 to 79	14.55%
80 to 89	32.86%
90 to 99	30.04%
100 to 109	8.92%
110 to 119	6.57%
120 and above	0.93%

However, a curve would allow us to better represent the distribution. I used the results from the British study of 15,000 men to draw the curve below. This study has two advantages over the one by Khérumian: It is more recent and is more representative, since it involves more people.

Here is the curve representing the distribution of size of penises in a flaccid state:

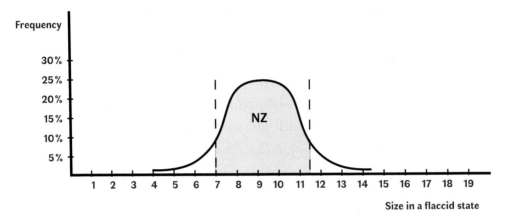

If we compare this graph to the IQ bell curve, we can begin to define a "normal zone," called NZ. Shown in gray, this zone represents the "common" or "ordinary" penises.

Here is the curve representing penis lengths when erect. Note that it is almost identical to the above curve, with a simple shift:

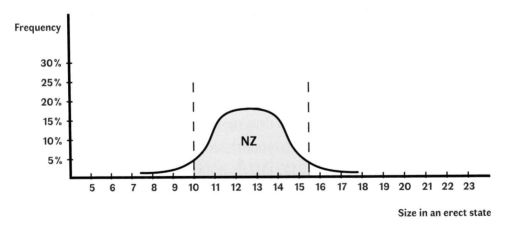

Here, too, we can begin to define a normal zone, also shown in gray. However, the choice of where to set boundaries is highly arbitrary and questionable. Some studies also consider the length of a stretched penis in a flaccid state. I did not include these studies here, since they do not provide any information of interest. In practice, the stretched length is the same as the length when erect.

Around 2 percent of men have a truly small penis, measuring less than 2.75 inches (7 cm) when erect — they have what is called a microphallus or micropenis. A later section is dedicated to this very real problem (see pages 57–59). Treatments, and they do exist, are outlined in the chapter dedicated to penis enlargement (see pages 61–75).

Most men have a penis measuring between 3.1 and 6.7 inches (8–17 cm) when erect, enough for penetration and a satisfying sex life. Reproduction is also possible, since sperm needs to be deposited at least 1.5 inches (4 cm) inside the entrance of the vagina in order to have a reasonable chance of passing through the cervix. Since sperm is ejaculated, it will thereby be in the right place.

Approximately 1 percent of men have a very large penis, measuring more than 5 inches (13 cm) when flaccid and more than 7 inches (18 cm) when erect. It is, of course, from this 1 percent that porn actors are recruited. However, that does not mean these well-endowed men will have a more satisfying sex life than others. In fact, a survey showed that when asked about their penis size, around 5 percent of men said they wished it were a little smaller. The same proportion of women, 5 percent, said they wished their partners had a smaller penis.

Here I offer you a relevant anecdote from my professional practice. Several years ago, a 50-something-year-old female patient who was married and had just returned from a one-week solo getaway at a resort in Sicily told me about this experience (sometimes you hear unexpected things during a consultation). She'd met an Italian man there, and that evening, with the help of the ambiance and wine, she let herself be seduced and brought the man back to her suite. When she saw the erect penis of her soon-to-be partner, she took a step back thinking, "I'm going to have to stick it between my thighs…" The experience was painful, and it did not happen again.

Excess Weight and Penis Length

The apparent or visible length of the penis is considerably shorter in overweight men and shorter still in obese men. This is easily explained: In men, excess fat **(1)** tends to accumulate around the midsection, which

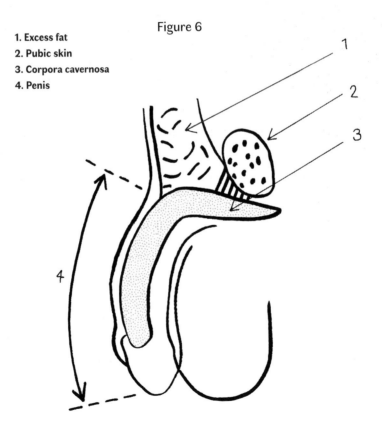

Figure 6

1. Excess fat
2. Pubic skin
3. Corpora cavernosa
4. Penis

stretches the pubic skin (2). The visible part of the corpora cavernosa (3) is thereby reduced, which makes the penis look shorter (4). This phenomenon is called a "buried penis."

Size by Ethnic Origin

In their studies, Khérumian and Juster cite the results of several earlier studies, which provide the following data for length by ethnic origin:

- Tonkinese: 2.91 inches (74 mm)
- Fuegian: 3.03 inches (77 mm)
- Japanese: 3.39 (86 mm)
- European: 3.54–3.94 inches (90–100 mm)
- Mandja (African): 4.29 inches (109 mm)
- Sara (African): 4.88 inches (124 mm)

Regarding the last two measurements, Khérumian observed that Stigler (published in 1943) thought that the long and thick aspect of the penis of certain African races is partly due to their foreskin, which Stigler describes as being extraordinarily long and thick.

Khérumian also noted that Stigler observed that the penises of African men tend to be larger in a flaccid state than the penises of European men but are proportionally smaller when erect.

More recently, a study published in 2012 in *Personality and Individual Differences* and led by Richard Lynn, a former professor emeritus of psychology at Ulster University in North Ireland, investigated the average length of penises by ethnic origin. Here are the results, in ascending order:

- Korea (both combined): 3.3 inches (9.652 cm)
- France: 5.3 inches (13.462 cm)
- Sweden: 5.9 inches (14.986 cm)
- Italy: 6.2 inches (15.748 cm)
- Iceland: 6.5 inches (16.51 cm)
- Congo: 7.1 inches (18.034 cm)

Remember, however, that there can be significant variations between individuals of the same ethnicity, as shown in the two studies reviewed at the beginning of this chapter (see pages 40–43), and it is, of course, not possible to estimate an individual's penis size based on their ethnic origin. At most, trends can be derived from the data.

Statistically, Asians have smaller penises than Europeans, who themselves have smaller penises than Africans.

Let's conclude with David Parirenyatwa, a former Zimbabwean health minister and the author of a report on the use of condoms in his country in the fight against the AIDS virus. He writes:

Youths now have a particular condom that they like, but we don't manufacture them. We import condoms from China and some men complain they are too small.

What About Kids?

At birth, the penis generally measures between 0.5 and 1.5 inches (1.5–3.5 cm). However, the length may be difficult to assess because of the common presence of a long foreskin. Throughout infancy and childhood, size increases, but it rarely exceeds 2 to 2.75 inches (5–7 cm) by the age of 10 years, i.e., right before puberty. Among heavier boys, fat in the pelvic region can give the impression that the penis is shorter due to "buried penis," as with adults.

The hormone testosterone is released in large quantity by the testicles during puberty, and this hormonal surge leads to spectacular changes: the voice deepens, the musculature develops, and hair appears on the pubis, armpits and face. Penis size increases as well, and, in general, it reaches its adult size at around 16 to 17 years of age.

When a truly small penis is identified during childhood, it is possible to improve the situation by administering testosterone, generally through intramuscular injections of a long-acting drug (which helps space out the injections, which generally don't go over very well at that age). This hormone is effective during infancy and childhood but less so once puberty begins. Furthermore, if too much is administered or for too long, testosterone accelerates bone maturation, which results in a small stature in adulthood.

A Few Remarkable Penises

Rasputin

Rasputin was born in Siberia in 1869. He first had sex at the age of 13, when he lost his virginity in a banya, the famous Russian steam baths, to a beautiful widow who is only remembered by her first name, Maria.

During that time, Russia was ruled by Czar Nicholas II, whose son Alexei suffered from hemophilia. Rasputin, then 36 years old, presented himself as a healer and visited the imperial court to reduce the intensity of the boy's attacks, apparently through prayers and the laying on of hands.

In reality, his actions simply interrupted the remedy being given to the czarevitch to relieve his pain: aspirin. Back then, the medication was well known for its pain-relieving effects, but nothing was known about its anticoagulant properties, which would only have worsened the extent of Alexei's hemorrhaging.

As a very prominent man whose company was sought after, Rasputin gave free rein to his sexuality, and there are dozens, even hundreds, of women who participated in his many orgies. The rumor at the time was that he had a 12-inch (30 cm) long penis when erect and could have sex 10 times in a row.

However, the prominence he gained in the imperial court did not please everyone, and his dead body was found floating in the Neva River in December 1916. A servant who helped retrieve the body took advantage of a moment when the rescuers were distracted and severed Rasputin's penis and snatched it. No one knows what then happened to it.

According to some rumors, it was found in Paris after the Bolshevik Revolution, and this relic was allegedly adored by Russian women in exile who sought to remedy infertility. Between the two World Wars, a London auction house offered it to the highest bidder, but the object turned out to be a sea cucumber. These days, the museum of erotica in St. Petersburg displays a jar containing a 11.2 inch (28.5 cm) long penis preserved in formalin and presented as being Rasputin's, but it is actually the penis of a baby elephant.

Henri de Toulouse-Lautrec

Henri de Toulouse-Lautrec (1864–1901) lived at La Fleur blanche, a famous Parisian brothel. The painter suffered from pycnodysostosis, which is a genetic disease that was likely caused by his parents' inbreeding. It causes spontaneous fractures and a small stature. He also had a significantly large penis and priapism. The contrast between the artist's small size and his oversized penis, which was erect most of the time, led to the nickname "the tea pot," given to him by some of the prostitutes he frequented. Other boarders at La Fleur blanche called him "the scout" because, just like them, he was always prepared.

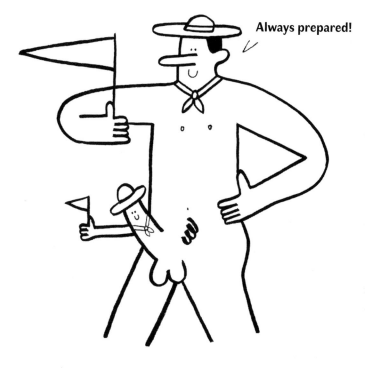

Always prepared!

Jonah Falcon

American Jonah Falcon was briefly famous in July 2012, when newspapers around the world reported his mishap. Falcon was stopped at the San Francisco International Airport because police noticed a suspicious protrusion in his pants. Upon closer inspection, they discovered that it was not a concealed bomb but the suspect's penis. A good-sized member, measuring 9.4 inches (24 cm) when flaccid and 13.4 inches (34 cm) when erect (34.29 cm). Despite the offers that poured in after the various reports about him, Falcon has always refused to appear in porn.

Roberto Esquivel Cabrera

Roberto Esquivel Cabrera requested disability payments from the Mexican government stating that his penis measuring 48.21 cm (which is 18.98 inches) prevented him from working. After medical verification, the measurement was amended to a more modest length of 5.9 inches (15 cm); the remainder was only a very long foreskin. It all made sense once the candidate for the world's longest penis acknowledged that he had, over years, suspended weights from his penis to elongate it. He had only succeeded in stretching his foreskin in excess of 12 inches (30 cm).

Long Dong Silver

Dong, as you likely know, is slang for penis. Long Dong Silver is a porn star who became famous in the late 1970s, mainly due to his penis, which measured a respectable 18 inches (45.7 cm) long when erect. Recently, photographer Jay Myrdal revealed that the erect penis of Long Dong Silver is actually "only" 9 inches (23 cm). The extra 9 inches (23 cm) came from a carefully glued latex prosthesis made by Christopher Tucker, the same man who created the makeup effects to transform John Hurt in *The Elephant Man*. Now we understand how Long Dong Silver was able to tie his penis in a knot...

Rocco Siffredi

During his childhood, Rocco Siffredi, born in the small Italian village of Ortona, was an altar boy, and his mother intended for him to become a priest. However, he had a different destiny. From the age of 10, he displayed sexual compulsion and masturbated all day long. In a 2016 interview, he said his penis was a demon that took control of his body.

With a 9-inch (23 cm) long penis when erect, he has used it extensively in different ways and shown it off in no less than 1,500 porn movies, filmed with 5,000 partners. Rocco Siffredi is known as the "Italian Stallion."

The Microphallus

Conventionally, a microphallus, also called micropenis, measures less than 1.6 inches (4 cm) when flaccid and less than 2.75 inches (7 cm) when erect. Statistically, less than 2 percent of penises fall into this category.

Napoleon was a big man in politics and military matters, but some of his other measurements were quite modest. In 1821, his personal physician, Francesco Antommarchi, performed an autopsy on his illustrious patient, assisted by seven British doctors. He mentions in *The Last Days of Napoleon: Memoirs of the Last Two Years of Napoleon's Exile* that the imperial penis measured 1.5 inches (3.8 cm). Antommarchi removed several of Napoleon's organs, including his heart and stomach, which were submerged into a jar filled with alcohol. He also removed his penis, which underwent a journey that few other penises could claim. The famous organ was given to Abbot

Vignali, who administered the last sacraments to the emperor and remained with the family until 1916. At that time, it was bought by an Englishman, who sold it eight years later for the sum of £400 (equivalent to nearly $32,000 today!) to an American named Rosenbach. Some 60 years later, it was bought by an American urologist from New Jersey named John K. Lattimer. Currently, the daughter of this doctor, named Evan, keeps the relic in her house in Englewood and refuses to show it.

————

Let's now return to our era. Doctors have noted that, since the 1990s, microphalluses are increasingly common. This is probably due to the growing presence of endocrine disruptors in our environment. These chemical substances are called hormone mimetics. In plain language, this means that they possess hormonal properties and can be active in very small amounts. Bisphenol A is the most common among them, but there are dozens. They are also associated with other harmful effects, such as triggering puberty earlier and earlier in females, increasing the rates of testicular cancer in developed countries and lowering sperm quality.

It's possible, to some extent, to increase the size of a microphallus. The procedures are discussed in the chapter dedicated to increasing penis size (see pages 61–75).

At one time, every year in June, a bar in Brooklyn organized a pageant for the smallest penis. Competitors paraded, naked, in front of a jury. A total of $200 and a scepter (equipped with a magnifying glass) was given to the winner. The winner of the 2013 parade commented:

The size of a man's penis does not matter for who he is as a person or in a relationship. Same thing with breast size. We're all made in different shapes and sizes, but the media puts pressure on people to look a certain way. Most people do not look that way. Some people let that false sense of body image upset them and they shouldn't be upset at all.

In the 1960s and 1970s, a certain number of boys born with a microphallus, particularly in the United States, were operated on very early in life and transformed into girls. Surgeons removed these boys' testicles, fashioned a clitoris out of their glans penis and created a neovagina.

These children were then raised as girls. The practice of forced sex reassignment is, however, completely reprehensible and was abandoned.

The Manning Index

The Manning Index reflects a fetus's exposure to androgens (male hormones) in utero. It is calculated simply by dividing the length of the index finger on the right hand by the length of the ring finger on the same hand. The lower the ratio, the higher the exposure to androgens. In females, these two fingers are generally the same length, and the Manning Index is close to 1. In males, the ring finger is generally longer, and the Manning Index on average is lower than 1.

Penis size is largely influenced by this prenatal exposure to hormones; therefore, it is possible to predict, to a certain extent, the length of a man's penis by looking at his hand. All you need to do is lay it flat. If the ring finger is longer than the index finger, the man has a small penis. If, on the contrary, the index finger is longer, the penis is too. (Now there's a way to keep things interesting at your next office party!)

The Manning Index can also be low in other circumstances, such as in those who suffer from Asperger's syndrome, an autism spectrum disorder that is not generally associated with intellectual disability and is sometimes associated with extraordinary abilities. Autism is linked to a number of factors. Some are genetic and others are environmental, but they are not widely understood, and it is possible that a fetus being exposed to low levels of androgen hormones plays a role. An exposure to endocrine disruptors has also been suggested as a possible cause.

How To Increase Penis Size

"Oh Father," said a little frog to the big one sitting by the side of a pool. "I have seen such a terrible monster! It was big as a mountain, with horns on its head, and a long tail, and it had hoofs divided in two."

"Tush, child, tush," said the old frog, "that was only farmer White's ox. It isn't so big either; he may be a little bit taller than I, but I could easily make myself quite as broad; just you see."

So he blew himself out, and blew himself out, and blew himself out.

"Was he as big as that?" he asked.

"Oh, much bigger than that," said the young frog.
— Aesop, The Frog and the Ox

Many procedures have been proposed to increase penis size, which is hardly surprising when you know that 45 percent of the male population feel they are not well-endowed and wish they had a bigger penis. Some methods are ancient and traditional, while others are more recent and modern. But if you're so inclined, which one should you choose? And what should you expect? We will dive deeper into those points, but first we will explore the recognized medical recommendations.

When Is Penis Enlargement Medically Justified?

The Microphallus

Only a true microphallus is justified for treatment to enlarge it. There is no real consensus, but it is generally not considered justified to treat a penis that is smaller than 1.5 inches (4 cm) when flaccid state and 2.75 inches (7 cm) when erect. A penis of 2.75 inches (7 cm) when erect is, of course, not large and its owner may never be a porn star, but it can certainly give pleasure to his partner, and if the end goal of the sexual encounter is procreation, penis size is less relevant than the expulsion of semen during ejaculation. The semen will be deposited far enough into the vagina to allow the sperm to reach the cervix.

If the microphallus is taken care of before puberty, the treatment of choice is the administration of testosterone. In this case, the hormone is generally administered by injections. It will make the penis grow in length as well as cause other bodily changes in the boy: increase musculature, hair growth (pubis, armpits, face) and a change in voice. Another effect is the fusion of epiphyseal plates. These plates are areas of bones that allow them to grow, hence their other name, growth plates. Once these plates ossify, growth stops. Therefore, testosterone should be handled with care: enough to be effective, but not so much as to impede growth.

After puberty, it is useless to administer testosterone; it will not change the penis's length, whatever the dosage or method of administration. Other procedures are required.

Other Cases

The proliferation of pornography, particularly on the Internet, can all too easily distort a person's view of themselves and their sexuality. According to Dr. Paolo Gontero, a urologist in Turin and the author of a well-documented work on the methods of lengthening the penis, many men who consult him for penis enlargement are in the normal range for length, and it is enough to show them photos of "normal" penises to reassure them and dissuade them from pursuing any procedure. However, there are men who suffer from penile dysmorphic disorder, and they remain convinced that their penis is too small. For these men, psychological care is likely to be more beneficial than a surgical procedure.

Dietary Supplements

I collected the names of ingredients in various dietary supplements that claim to increase penis size. They include:

- Vitamins (B6, C, Niacin, Riboflavin and Thiamin).
- Amino acids, including taurine and arginine, among others. Taurine is, with caffeine, one of the main components of a well-known energy drink. It prevents you from sleeping, thus lengthening your period of wakefulness — but nothing else!
- Mineral salts, such as magnesium.
- Plant extracts, like fenugreek, which will not add any inches but may add a few pounds, since it stimulates the appetite, promoting weight gain.

- Pumpkin seed extract. My great-grandmother, like all grandmothers and great-grandmothers, had her little household tips. She would collect her fingernail clippings and embed them in the soil of her pots as fertilizer. Another trick: she would set pumpkin seeds aside, not to enlarge my great-grandfather's penis but to treat intestinal worms. Pumpkin seeds are quite effective at removing pinworms, roundworms, and tapeworms.

In short, none of the supplements listed above is known to have any effect on penis size.

Other plants may also be found in dietary supplements, like maca, muira puama, *Tribulus terrestris*, hogweed and even damiana. These plants will not elongate your penis, but they are rumored to be aphrodisiacs that facilitate erection. In reality, they are far from having the effectiveness of Viagra, Cialis and similar medications.

Gels

In the famous Kama Sutra, Vatsyayana gives us a recipe intended to fatten up the "linga." Simply coat it with buffalo butter. Now all you have to do is make your way to a grocery store!

A website selling a gel to elongate the penis has shown real and uncommon honesty by specifying the product's ingredients, advising that the gel is safe and hypoallergenic because it is made with water.

Injections

Like everyone else, Thai people dream of having a good-sized penis, and in recent years, they have injected their members with different products to try to go from S to XL. Dr. Surat Kittisupaporn, a urologist in Bangkok, has unfortunately seen the catastrophic results of injecting olive oil, silicone, beeswax and paraffin into the penis. In the best cases, these products cause painful nodules. Often, especially when the injections are too deep and have excessively damaged the corpora cavernosa, the man can no longer get an erection. In the worst cases, when there is necrosis, the penis needs to be amputated.

The United States, meanwhile, has started a new biohacker trend. Simply put, biohackers look to improve the function of their body by using modern biology. One such person, Ben Greenfield, a sports coach, was injected with stem cells. The procedure took place at a biotechnology clinic in Florida. He started out happy with the results, but during an interview he added that he prefers not to take measurements.

Another product tested via injections is botulinum toxin. This product is currently used in cosmetic procedures to smooth out wrinkles and mask other damage caused by time. Botulinum toxin was proposed to prevent the exaggerated retraction of the penis, making it look smaller. There would thereby be a small improvement in the length of the flaccid penis.

Hyaluronic acid is another widely used product in cosmetic procedures. This product is natural and well-tolerated by the body. A little history: for a long time, this product was extracted from rooster combs. Hyaluronic acid injections can help fill in wrinkles on the face or reshape an area, such as the buttocks, thereby avoiding implants. Although this use is banned in the United States, some cosmetic surgeons use hyaluronic acid injections to increase the diameter of the penis. Results are sometimes disastrous, not only on an aesthetic level (deformations, nodules), but also on a functional level, causing erectile dysfunction. Several years ago, a man was (poorly) treated, not to say butchered, with hyaluronic acid by a Parisian surgeon who was said to specialize in "intimate" surgery for men, and he took that practitioner to court.

To wrap up the topic of injections, let us consider the Tupinambá people of Brazil. In the past, the men of this tribe would voluntarily let a snake bite their penis to increase its size. The bite was extremely painful and completely ineffective. According to some non-verified rumors, a Parisian surgeon who specialized in intimate surgery for men sought to diversify his practice and financed an expedition to bring specimens of the reptiles back to his clinic.

Weights

If you take a piece of modeling clay and gently pull on it, it will elongate and maintain its new length. It is probably a finding of this kind that has inspired some men to suspend weights from their penis to lengthen it. In India, the Naga Baba sect is well-known for two things. First, its members live naked, coated with the ashes from funeral pyres. Second, they reject sexuality and demonstrate this by rendering their penis inoperable. To do this, they attach heavier and heavier weights to their penis to lengthen it.

Travelers have stated seeing such genitals reach a length of almost 18 inches (45 cm), foreskin included. This procedure is effective, but let's remember that the goal is not to have the longest penis — it's to render it incapable of erection. This impotence is due to micro-lesions in various structures in the penis (corpora cavernosa, vessels, nerves), which are caused by the forced lengthening.

There are modern versions of this procedure. One needs to tie weights to one's penis (the load can be by increments of 10 ounces or 250 g) and sit with one's legs spread open, the penis hanging and pulling downward. It is necessary to stay like this for several hours. The website touting this method recommends having reading materials or a smartphone handy.

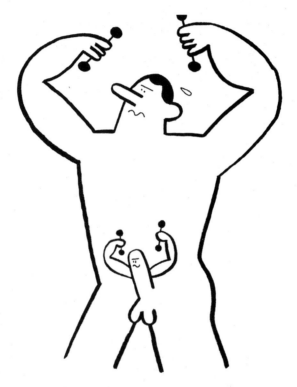

Extenders

This device consists of a part that supports the base of the penis and a movable part that goes around the tip of the penis. A spring helps separate these two pieces, which is supposed to passively lengthen the penis. Dr. Paolo Gontero, the previously mentioned associate professor of urology at the University of Turin, compiled a list of various studies on the results achieved with extenders. His work shows that this procedure has a certain level of effectiveness. A study was done in 2002 with a device, originating in Spain, under the brand name Andropenis. This device was worn on average six hours per day, and after four months, the gain in length was on average 0.71 inches (1.8 cm) with extremes of 0.2 inches (0.5 cm) and 1.22 inches (3.1 cm). Another study conducted with the same device had subjects wear it for four hours per day for six months. They achieved a lengthening of 0.67 to 0.9 inches (1.7–2.3 cm). However, in both of those studies, there was no increase in diameter. Photos of the Andropenis show a large device that would be impossible to conceal in pants. It is likely that these stretches were done in the evening, at home, unless it was worn at night. There are many knockoffs of this device. It is worth noting that there is a similar device said to correct penile curvature caused by Peyronie's disease, which has mixed results. Despite Dr. Gontero's optimistic conclusions, you must be careful with any such product. Like with the weights, extenders work by stretching the penis, and it is possible that the disadvantages are the same in the long run.

Pumps

Also called vacuums, these devices are made up of a cylinder connected at one end to a pump that sucks air. The penis is inserted into the other end, and the vacuum created in the clylinder causes it to swell.

Such devices are promoted as a treatment for erectile dysfunction as well as to increase penis size. However, if the penis does gain a little extra length immediately afterward, it quickly reverts to its original size.

Surgery

Three types of surgical procedures are offered in current practice: liposuction of prepubic fat, penoplasty to lengthen the penis and penoplasty to thicken the penis. Two other surgical procedures look promising, but there is not yet enough information available to properly assess them.

Liposuction of Prepubic Fat

This procedure consists of sucking the fat found in front of the pubis, which is responsible for the "buried penis" phenomenon in overweight men. To illustrate, here are two penis drawings:

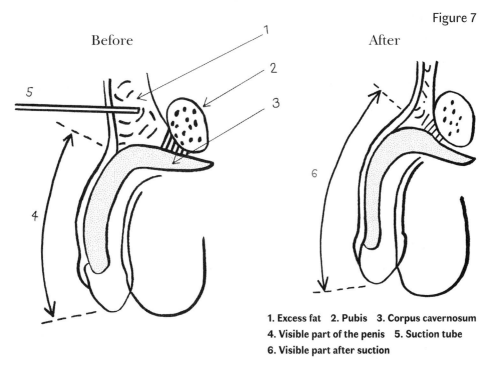

Figure 7

Before   After

1. Excess fat   2. Pubis   3. Corpus cavernosum
4. Visible part of the penis   5. Suction tube
6. Visible part after suction

We can see that a simple reduction in the amount of fat can help add an inch or so.

It is easy to determine whether you can benefit from this operation. Position a finger horizontally along your pubic region, just above the base of your penis, and press on the skin. If your finger clearly pushes back the skin and increases the visible part of your penis, you will likely benefit! You could also simply reduce your beer intake and go on a diet to lose weight. You will kill two birds with one stone: obtaining a longer penis and unburdening your liver.

Penoplasty for Lengthening

The corpora cavernosa are connected to the pubis by a ligament, known as the suspensory ligament of the penis. This ligament helps the penis point upward when erect. Ingenious surgeons came up with the idea of cutting it to let the penis hang a bit lower when flaccid, making it look longer. To prevent the ligament from "snapping back" to the pubis once its cut, the surgeon inserts a silicone prosthesis. Plastic surgery to lengthen the skin is performed to help the penis descend freely. Some commercial websites promise to lengthen the penis by a few inches. However, the actual gain is modest: 0.5 to 1 inch (1–2 cm) maximum and only when flaccid (the length when erect will stay exactly the same). Furthermore, as previously stated, the suspensory ligament of the penis helps the erect organ point upward. Once the ligament is cut, the erect penis will inevitably point downward and must be manually redirected before any attempt at penetration.

The diagram (opposite) shows a broad outline of the procedure.

This operation is performed around the world. According to statistics from the International Society of Aesthetic Plastic Surgery, demand for penoplasty for lengthening is high among Germans. In 2013, members of this learned society performed 15,414 such procedures around the world, 2,786 of which were in Germany.

Figure 8

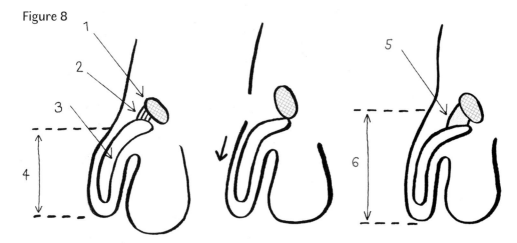

1. Pubic bone 2. Suspensory ligament 3. Corpus cavernosum 4. Apparent length before surgery
5. Silicone prosthesis 6. Apparent length after surgery

Penoplasty to Thicken

Some men are satisfied with the length of their penis but not the diameter. For them, plastic surgeons have come up with lipostructure. This procedure involves sucking fat from the abdominal region and reinjecting it under the skin of the penis. Thus, thickness is added. There is one benefit: The fat comes from the man being operated on himself, and it will therefore not be rejected.

However, this operation doesn't always provide the expected results. For starters, the fat must be spread evenly to avoid bumps. Afterward, there is an inevitable partial reabsorption of the fat, and the result is not final until after a few months. Swiss doctors are lucky enough to have a highly regarded journal, the *Revue Médicale Suisse* (Swiss medical review). A very serious study on techniques for increasing penis size appeared in its pages in 2004, and this article reports this loss varying between 30 percent and 90 percent. In other words, after several months, it is possible to be left with only 10 percent of the injected fat. Back to square one...

Risks

These operations are not without risks. Like all surgical procedures, they can lead to potentially serious complications. The most common of these is the unsightly appearance of the scar from penoplasty for lengthening, which is not always concealed under hair. According to an article in the previously mentioned *Revue Médicale Suisse*, half of men who underwent the procedure have one.

However, there are much more concerning issues. In early 2019, an extremely wealthy 65-year-old diamond dealer who got a penis enlargement in a specialized cosmetic clinic in Paris had a heart attack during surgery and could not be resuscitated.

Costs

Like many cosmetic surgeries, penis lengthening is not within the reach of everyone's budget. Clinics located abroad, such as in Central or South America, can have substantially lower prices. Specialized travel agents even offer packages combining the operation itself with a vacation. These offers should be considered with extreme caution, however. Even in cases when the surgeon and clinic are competent and professional, long-term follow-up care is often non-existent once you're back home, due to the travel distance required. In addition, if the procedure fails, you will have no recourse, and it will be impossible for you to have it redone or to be compensated.

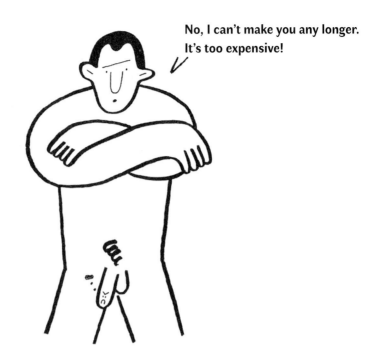

Two Promising Techniques

An innovative technique that truly lengthens the penis has just been developed. It consists of detaching the glans penis from the end of the corpora cavernosa, inserting a piece of rib cartilage and then reattaching the glans. Studies have shown that the piece of cartilage remains alive. Unlike conventional penoplasty, it is a true lengthening that will last. The researchers have published their results, which seem rather interesting. Here are the measurements of two men with microphalusses.

Subject 1

Before the procedure: length when flaccid 1.3 inches (3.2 cm)

                               length when erect 3.1 inches (7.9 cm)

After the procedure: length when flaccid 2.4 inches (6.1 cm)

                               length when erect 4.3 inches (10.8 cm)

Subject 2

Before the procedure: length when flaccid 1.0 inches (2.6 cm)

                               length when erect 2.6 inches (6.7 cm)

After the procedure: length when flaccid 2.2 inches (5.6 cm)

                               length when erect 3.7 inches (9.4 cm)

As this operation is new, it still needs to be assessed. A final verdict has yet to be determined.

Another new technique helps increase the diameter of the penis when erect. Furthermore, unlike fat injections, the results are definitive. It consists of splitting the tunica albuginea from the two corpora cavernosa lengthwise and then grafting a section of the saphenous vein along the length. This increases the diameter of each corpus cavernosum once it fills with blood (in other words, during an erection). In a flaccid state, the penis is the same size.

Patients who have undergone this procedure did not present any problems during their follow-ups, particularly no erectile dysfunction. Results are quite satisfactory, with an increase in diameter of 0.4 to 0.8 inches (1.1–2.1 cm).

Jelqing

Jelqing is a traditional method of lengthening the penis that is found in parts of Asia and the Middle East. It is a kind of massage for increasing blood flow in the penis to increase its length and thickness. A man holds his penis, which must be semi-erect, between the thumb and index of one hand, the two digits forming a ring. He then raises this rounded grip towards the tip of the penis to push blood toward the glans. This maneuver, which should be painless, is repeated hundreds of times a day. There is no study proving the effectiveness of jelqing; in fact, urologists caution against it, citing complications such as hematomas and fractures of the corpora cavernosa.

Pain, Discharge and Spots: Penis Problems

The penis can be subject to various difficulties, temporary problems, accidents and even occasional breakdowns.

It could be a defect, a trauma, a misplaced opening, an infection — your penis could even be stolen! How, you may ask? You will see, and it's very interesting.

To keep this chapter from simply becoming a list of horrors, I've included some anecdotes — consultations that were particularly memorable or entertaining. They're a bit like the doctor's version of the tall tales so common among fishermen and hunters, but instead of a huge fish or massive buck, it's an unlikely patient!.

These are stories that stand out from the many mundane consultations, such as a spot-on diagnosis of a rare disease made late at night, when you were so tired after having looked at 10 ear infections and refilling just as many prescriptions, but you had the right instincts and didn't miss even the smallest symptom. Or maybe you were called upon to examine a celebrity passing through town. Anything can become a true story or tall tale; it need only pop up in daily life.

I, too, have stories and tales related to our subject, which I will share with you for your edification and entertainment.

Penile Adhesions

In children, penile adhesions between the foreskin's mucous membrane and the base of the glans penis are common. They often worry mothers and are a frequent reason for doctors' visits. Until recently, doctors — both general practitioners and pediatricians — advising "releasing" these adhesions, using as much force as necessary. During my studies, I was taught the recommended way of releasing them. It involved sliding a small, ridged probe (a metal tool generally used for dissections) under the adhesions and then lifting them, with a bit of force, to detach them. Needless to say, young boys, so poorly treated, would reluctantly come for follow-ups.

It is now recommended to leave these adhesions alone. During adolescence, a boy's own nocturnal manual experiments at that age are enough to make them go away.

The male genital area secretes a whitish substance called smegma that tends to accumulate under penile adhesions. This accumulation can sometimes become quite smelly. This is a normal physiological process, and it should not prompt the release of these adhesions. A gentle pulling back of the foreskin followed by a simple wash with soap and water is generally enough to manage smegma. There is no need to use antiseptic products, as the glans penis has its own bacterial flora, called microbiota, that must be respected. The chapter dedicated to penis hygiene provides more information on smegma (see pages 186–189).

Agenesis of the Penis

Children with this rare abnormality (around one birth in 20 million) are born without a penis. Recently, Andrew Wardle, a British man born with this condition, was briefly famous in May 2018, when he received an artificial penis implant. The implant was made with tissues from one of his forearms. The bionic penis can even simulate an erection. The bionic penis is equipped with a pump and two flexible reservoirs, which the man can fill with saline solution. This operation and implant allowed the man to experience sex at the age of 45 years old. You can't stop progress!

Balanitis

This word's etymology provides insights into what this medical term means: *Balanos* means "glans" in Greek, and in medicine the suffix -itis generally means inflammation, as in osteitis (inflammation of the bones), urethritis (inflammation of the urethra), gastritis (inflammation of the stomach), gingivitis (inflammation of the gums) and so on.

The inflammation of the glans penis may have several origins:

- It is often caused by a bacterial infection.
- It can also result from a microscopic fungal infection, for example *Candida albicans*, a common fungus, which in that case is called a mycosis.
- Less often, it is caused by other things and can be a localized dermatological disease known to affect other parts of the body: lichen (dermatosis, not the plant), psoriasis, eczema, etc.
- Finally, and this is not uncommon, balanitis can be caused by excessive hygiene. In fact, while microbial and fungal balanitis

are often cause by lax hygiene habits, too rigorous hygiene habits can also create problems. We will review this in detail in the chapter dedicated to penis hygiene (see pages 186–189).

Let's end with a story from my practice... Some years ago, one of my patients came in for a consultation because his glans smelled like not-so-fresh fish. He indicated that this odor was only notice-able when soaping up. During the exam, his glans looked completely healthy: no redness, no visible lesions, no discharge from the meatus. The patient was a sensible person and not likely to complain about imaginary illnesses. Just in case, I recommended that he switch soaps. Sometime later, this man's partner came in for vulvitis, which is an irritation of the vulva.

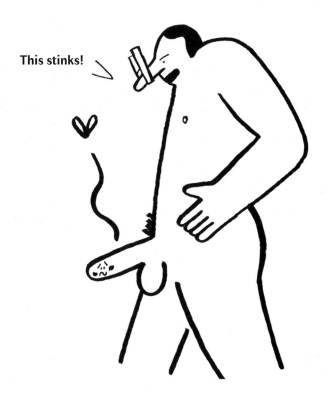

This stinks!

Since the clinical exam found only some normal discharge and I was not able to identify any possible bacteria, I requested a lab test with bacteriological testing. The bacteria *Gardnerella vaginalis* was identified.

Gardnerella vaginalis is known to emit a fishlike smell when it comes in contact with potassium, and this test is aptly called a "whiff test." This meant that the woman's partner was a healthy carrier of *Gardenella*, and when he applied soap, which is alkaline like potassium, to his penis, it released this strong fish smell. We don't always think of everything!

Cancer

Penile cancer is rare in Western countries. It is estimated that it only represents 0.6 percent of male cancers. The frequency is much higher in other parts of the world, particularly Africa and Brazil, where it represents 17 percent of tumors.

Several risk factors have been identified, including a lack of hygiene, local trauma and human papillomavirus (HPV) infection. Penile cancer is rare in men under 50 years old.

The glans and foreskin are most affected. Localization on the penis shaft is less common. This cancer can take the form of an ulcer, induration (i.e., hardening), persistent rash or even a localized thickening. Its progression is generally slow: It starts off locally, and it can then spread to the inguinal lymph nodes.

Depending on the degree of progression, treatment can include chemotherapy, radiation therapy or surgery.

Preventative measures may include circumcision (it has been shown that circumcised men are less affected) and the HPV vaccine.

Syphilis

Once referred to as the "great pox," syphilis was also often associated with particular cultures: The Italians, Germans and British called it the French disease, the French referred to it as the Neapolitan disease, the Russians named it the Polish disease, the Polish called it the German disease and the Turks called it the Christian disease. These various monikers, however, had more to do with politics than disease spread...

There are two main theories surrounding syphilis's origins. Researchers once posited that it was brought from the Americas to Europe by returning sailors who were part of Christopher Columbus's expedition. Newer evidence is suggesting different strains have existed on both continents for centuries, long before Columbus set sail.

Before the introduction of effective antibiotics, syphilis was a very common disease. Many famous men are said to have suffered from syphilis. They include the writers Charles Baudelaire, Gustave Flaubert, Guy de Maupassant and Oscar Wilde; painters Paul Gauguin and Vincent Van Gogh; rulers Henry VIII and Czar Ivan IV (Ivan the terrible); as well as famous Chicago gangster Al Capone.

In women, syphilitic chancres are generally found on the vulva or vagina. Illustrious women who are said to have suffered from the disease include author Karen Blixen and Hannah Chaplin, mother of Charlie Chaplin.

Treatment prior to the early 20th century was based on the administration of mercury, which was both dangerous and ineffective. It wasn't until after World War II, with the arrival of penicillin, that doctors were able to effectively treat it. This sexually transmitted disease then became very rare in Western countries, but it has made a comeback in the 2000s. Due to joint contaminated risk factors, it is now often associated with HIV infection.

Infection occurs through lesions containing the syphilis-causing bacteria, which is called *Treponema pallidum*. It can be a genital, oral or anal infection. In the early stages of the disease, one to three weeks after contact, an inoculation chancre appears (the term "inoculation" in this context means at the site of the infection). This lesion typically appears as a painless, pinkish round ulcer with an indurated (i.e., hard) base.

In males, the chancre is most commonly found on the shaft of the penis or the glans penis. An adenopathy (swelling of the lymph nodes) is often found in the groin. Adenopathies usually only affect a single lymph node.

In females, the chancre can be visible or hidden deeper inside the body, for example, in the vagina or uterus, where it can go unnoticed. If it is external, for example on the labia, it is often accompanied by inguinal adenopathy (i.e., inflammation of the lymph nodes in the groin).

A diagnosis is confirmed by a blood test. After its initial onset, the chancre disappears within a few weeks, even without treatment, but that doesn't mean that the *Treponema pallidum* bacterium is gone. The bacteria grow in the body and can spread to multiple organs.

There are very effective antibiotic treatments for syphilis. The one that is recommended — because it is the most effective, the best tolerated and the least expensive — is derived from penicillin. If the patient is allergic to penicillin a different drug is prescribed, most likely an antibiotic in the cycline family. If such a treatment is administered at the right time, *Treponema pallidum* disappears and healing is guaranteed. Without treatment, syphilis will evolve. A few months after the early stage, highly contagious lesions appear on mucous membranes and on the skin all over the body. Within a few years, *Treponema pallidum* can seriously damage the nervous system, joints and even the heart.

Throughout my career, I have only seen two chancres. The first one was on a truck driver who had a pricey encounter in a parking lot. He had a typical lesion. The second case, also typical, involved a young man who took part in sex tourism. In both cases, the infection was due to unprotected vaginal sex. Remember, however, that syphilis is also easily transmitted by fellatio (i.e., oral sex). Some years ago, I interviewed an elegant older woman to fill out her medical file. When I asked her what diseases she had had, she mentioned tonsilitis and then backtracked and said to me, "It wasn't really tonsilitis, it was…" She paused to think and then said, "It's coming back to me now. It was tonsillar syphilis."

Genital Warts

Infection by HPV (human papillomavirus) types 6 and 11 is likely to cause the appearance of sometimes very large growths on the skin or mucous membranes. These lesions are called condylomata or, more commonly, genital warts. They may also be referred to as "cockscomb" warts due to their resemblance to that part of a rooster. They are benign but highly contagious. Such warts can develop into cancer, but this is rare.

HPVs are easily transmitted from person to person through sex, but they can also be transmitted indirectly by, for example sharing a towel, or even through contact with a soiled surface (such as a bench in a sauna).

Warts are common on the genitals and anus, in both men and women. In men, they particularly affect the base of the glans penis and the inside of the foreskin, where they can form clusters.

In the section on penile cancer, we note that HPVs are often involved in this disease. Preventative measures, particularly vaccines, are therefore recommended for young people. There is currently only one vaccine available in the United States to protect against HPV. Gardasil 9 protects both males and females against seven types of HPV that cause cancer, including types 16 and 18, as well as types 6 and 11, which cause genital warts. Two other vaccines are available in Canada, Cervarix and Gardasil. Cervarix protects females against HPV types 16 and 18, while Gardasil protects both males and females against HPV types 6, 11, 16 and 18. Gardasil 9 is also available in Canada.

Genital warts are diagnosed visually. The physician may be able to reveal the affected areas with acetic acid dyes and the help of a magnifying glass. The affected areas will turn white.

Treatment consists of destroying the warts, most often by electrocautery, liquid nitrogen, laser treatment or a topical treatment such as imiquimod, podophyllin or trichloroacetic acid.

Sunburn

The penis's skin contains melanocytes, which are cells that secrete melanin and allow a person to tan. However, the skin in the genital area is very thin, particularly fragile and is only rarely or never exposed to the sun's rays. A tanning session, therefore, quickly risks turning into a sunburn. If you want to tan your whole body, you need to take some precautions. These are well-known, but it doesn't hurt to be reminded:

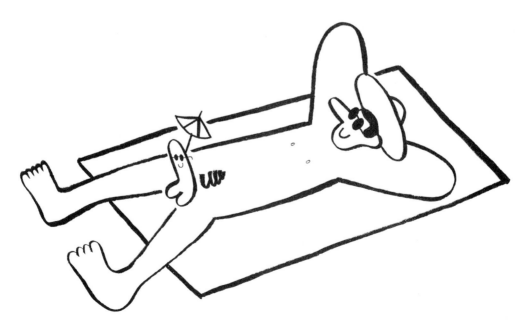

- Use a sunscreen with a high SPF.
- Avoid exposure between noon and 4 p.m.
- Tan gradually.

Congenital Curvature

This morphological (i.e., related to shape or form) anomaly is only visible when the penis is erect. The penis can be abnormally curved in two ways:
- The curvature can be ventral (i.e., along the bottom), which makes the glans point down, or
- the curvature can be lateral (i.e., along the side), which makes the penis point right or left.

If the curvature is not very significant, it mainly affects how the penis looks and how the person feels about it. When the deformity is more pronounced, it can cause difficulties with penetration during sex. Treatment, when necessary, is surgical and done during puberty. In the case of related hypospadias (see pages 91–93), treatment is generally done earlier. Surgical outcomes are often good and achieve satisfactory results. It should be mentioned that in most cases this treatment leads to a shortening of the penis by 0.5 to 1 inches (1–2 cm).

Diphallia

Diphallia is an extremely rare condition that affects males and creates two penises. The cause is unknown, but environmental factors, particularly endocrine disruptors, are suspected.

This anomaly is generally associated with other major defects in the urinary system or intestines. One of the two organs is usually rudimentary, meaning it is not functional, but there are exceptional cases of men who have two full-sized functional penises. One such case recently ended up all over the Internet. The man in question, nicknamed the Double Dick Dude, leveraged his anatomical particularity by making porn videos.

Elephantiasis

During my studies, I took a course on parasitology. During one of my classes, the professor showed a slide that is surely burned into the memory of every student who was present that day. The slide showed a man holding a wheelbarrow in which he had deposited his enormous testicles and penis. The collection was the size of a large pumpkin. This monstrosity was elephantiasis caused by a parasitic disease transmitted by mosquitos, called Bancroftian filariasis. The parasite obstructs the lymphatic vessels so that lymph infiltrates the skin, causing this monstrous swelling.

Epispadias

In this malformation, the urethra opens at the top of the penis. The opening can be situated near the pubis, on the dorsal side (top) of the penis or even on the glans penis. In the latter case, epispadias can go unnoticed for a long time if the opening is covered by the foreskin.

This condition is quite rare and is often linked to a malformation of the bladder. The cause is unknown. There are continent and incontinent forms of epispadias, depending on whether the bladder's sphincter is involved. When there is an associated bladder malformation, there is a risk of bladder cancer in adulthood. Treatment is surgical, generally done in the first months of life and consists of reconstructing a urethra and having it open on the ventral (under) side of the penis.

Fractures

Although it is not a bone, the penis can fracture. This accident can only occur when the penis is rigid, that is, during an erection. Fractures generally happen during sex that's a little too energetic (but not always, as we'll see later). It is a kind of sexual misstep, whereby an unfortunate fellow inadvertently disengages from his partner during the back-and-forth movements and then tries to reinsert it forcefully, has poor aim and then impacts his partner's perineum. The concerned party will feel a sharp crack, his partner as well, localized pain occurs, and his erection will go down (the medical term for this is detumescence). The penis becomes deformed due to swelling from a hematoma where the fracture occurred. This generally occurs at the base of the penis, and one corpus cavernosum is usually injured.

In the chapter dedicated to anatomy (see pages 12–21), we saw that the penis becomes rigid during an erection when blood fills the corpora cavernosa, which are contained in an envelope called the tunica albuginea. When the penis is fractured, the tunica albuginea ruptures, and blood leaves the injured corpus cavernosum and spreads under the skin, forming a hematoma. It's possible for the urethra to rupture as well; in that case, there will be a discharge of blood from the meatus.

You may wonder whether certain sexual positions are riskier than others. Urologists from the University of Campinas in Brazil asked that very question and conducted a study, which appeared in the *Advances of Urology* journal. We learn from that article that in 44 men who sustained a penis fracture, 12 were due to excessively rough handling, and 32 occurred during sex. Their results showed that the most dangerous position is with the partner on top (16 cases), followed by "doggy" style (eight cases). The good old missionary position seems the least risky, since it was responsible for only six cases.

Earlier I wrote that penile fractures don't always happen during sex. In fact, a dangerous practice called *taghaandan* consists of violently handling the penis to stop morning erections. It involves roughly bending and pressing it down. In this case, the fracture usually occurs in the upper section of the roughed-up penis.

With those cases, penis fractures are clinically diagnosed and are generally obvious to the naked eye. If there is doubt, the doctor can perform an ultrasound. Penis fractures are treated surgically, and the surgery is usually performed as an emergency procedure under general anesthesia. The surgeon makes a circular incision in the skin just below the glans penis and rolls up the skin, uncovering the penis, exposing the

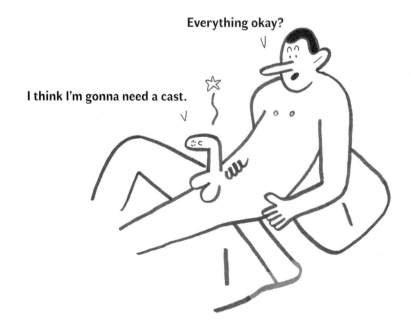

corpora cavernosa. Once the surgeon identifies the lesion, they suture the tunica albuginea with a dissolvable stitch. Some surgeons make a simple opening an inch or so long in the injured area and suture the tunica albuginea after draining the pool of blood. A ruptured urethra can also be surgically repaired.

In all cases, the patient must abstain from any form of sex for eight weeks. Complications are possible but rare. They include deformation, erectile dysfunction or even relapse of the fracture.

Scabies

Scabies is a contagious condition caused by a very small 0.008 to 0.01 inches (0.2 to 0.35 mm) mite called *Sarcoptes scabiei hominis*. This parasite can live on a person's skin. These mites dig tunnels while feeding on skin debris. Their presence and especially their droppings in the skin can lead to itching, which triggers scratching. Typically, the itching is more pronounced in the evening and at night. The areas of the body that are most likely to be affected include the sides of the fingers, the wrists, the buttocks and the genitals. The face is usually spared, except in infants. Transmissions typically occur through direct contact and more rarely through linens or clothing. Because of the possibility of spread during sex, by the proximity of the couple's epidermises, some doctors consider scabies a sexually transmitted disease.

Local scabies infestations at the penis are common and result in severe pruritus (a medical term for itching). The infested person will react by scratching, which can lead to local redness and excoriation (skin picking), which may become complicated by a secondary bacterial infection, which can then lead to impetigo, which is a superficial skin infection.

Diagnosis is clinical; it can be confirmed by examining samples under a microscope to find *Sarcoptes scabiei hominis*. The doctor may confirm the diagnosis by visually examining the patient using a magnifying glass, revealing the outlines of the tunnels created by the mites, which end with tiny protrusions. Treatment is generally local and involves repeated applications of a topical cream or lotion. There are also oral treatments, which I think are far more practical.

Frostbite

People who live in cold climates know this risk all too well; to urinate, they only let out the bare minimum of their penis to the open air. In fact, in very low temperatures, the penis can freeze in less than a minute, especially if it's windy. If there is no immediate care, a frostbitten penis can devolve into gangrene and loss of the organ. Some years ago, British newspapers amused their readers with reports of the misadventure of Kenneth Guillespie. This 64-year-old former mailman had very drunkenly attempted to "violate" a snowman and found himself in the hospital to receive treatment for his penis, which was frozen from the "coupling."

Herpes

Genital herpes is a highly contagious sexually transmitted infection. It is caused by herpes simplex virus type 2 (HSV-2). Another type of herpes virus (HSV-1) causes oral herpes, also called cold sores. However, oral-genital sex (fellatio, cunnilingus) can easily transmit HSV-1 to the genitals or HSV-2 from the genitals to the mouth. Both viruses cause the same disorders.

A herpes infection results in local pain, like stinging or burning, which precedes the appearance of vesicles (i.e., tiny blisters) that form in clusters. These vesicles then become small sores. A ganglion (a medical term for a swelling) may appear in the groin, damaging the genitals. The flare-up will seem to heal spontaneously in 8 to 10 days, but this is misleading. Once infected, the body cannot get rid of herpes, even with treatment.

The virus remains in the body, and the disease progresses into more or less frequent flare-ups. People who have many flare-ups one after the other can suffer greatly. Fatigue and exposure to the sun can trigger herpes flare-ups.

Treatment can be local or general. Topical products (creams, gels) are generally more effective. The most commonly prescribed treatment is valaciclover, sold under the brand name Valtrex.

Herpes can cause lesions all over the body, including the anus. This brings to mind another story from my practice.

Many years ago, I examined a young woman with anal herpes. When I told her the diagnosis, she told me, "I haven't had…," and she left out the final words, probably out of embarrassment. She was right though. It was not necessary for her to have had anal sex to suffer from a herpes lesion in that area. A simple contact is enough, such as a touch from a finger carrying the virus or discharge containing the virus coming into contact with another part of the body. There is also no need for a lesion; the herpes virus can take root on completely healthy skin.

Hypospadias

In epispadias, the urethra opens on top of the penis; in hypospadias, the urethra opens on the underside of the penis. The term "hypospadias" is formed from two Greek words: *hypo*, which means "under," and *spadias*, which means "opening."

This malformation affects around one in 300 males, but its incidence has doubled in the last 40-some years. The opening can be near the tip of the penis or, less commonly, in the middle or even close to the base. It is sometimes, but rarely, associated with other urinary or genital malformations.

Causes of hypospadias are still not well-known. In some cases, there is a genetic factor, in which case the malformation can run in families. However, these forms represent less than 10 percent of cases. Other contributing factors include twinship and substances a mother consumes during her pregnancy. For example, certain medications have been linked to hypospadias, particularly sodium valproate, as have certain foods, particularly those that contain phytoestrogens, which are analogs of the female hormone estrogen. Soy is a rich source of phytoestrogens. Other substances strongly linked to hypospadias include certain pesticides, cosmetics, hair dyes and even bisphenol A (BPA). These products contain endocrine disruptors, which are increasingly widespread in our environment, hence the increase in hypospadias cases (and many other health problems).

One well-established cause is a medication, and its effects can be transgenerational. I am referring to DES (or diethylstilbestrol). This hormone was prescribed to pregnant women from the 1940s to the 1970s to prevent spontaneous abortions. It was later banned, when it was found that "DES daughters," a term that refers to women who were exposed to the drug in utero, frequently had a rare type of vaginal cancer. The harmful effects of this medication also continued to affect males of the next generation, who were the grandsons of the women originally treated. The frequency of hypospadias in these males is 20 times higher than the general population.

Hypospadias affects both the urinary and the reproductive functions. In the urinary system, whereby the urethra's opening is far from the meatus, the affected male must urinate sitting down. Some patients have a hard time with this, as they think the seated position is reserved for females. However, there is not a "manly" way to pee and a "girly" way to pee. Urinating in a seated position is in no way a reflection of who a person is.

In the reproductive system, hypospadias leads to the sperm needing to travel a greater distance to reach the cervix, since the urethral opening is further down the penis. In order to have the greatest chance at fertilizing an egg, the sperm must reach the cervix, so hypospadias can lead to infertility.

Treatment is surgical and involves reconstructing the urethra and bringing it as close as possible to its correct anatomical position. Complications are rare but include the appearance of a fistula along the pathway of the new urethra. The current trend is to operate when the child is around one year old. However, each case is assessed individually, and there is no need to rush to go under the knife. For several years, I followed a man with hypospadias whose opening was high enough and who did not have an operation. He lived a perfectly normal life, had kids, and told me that he urinated like the average Joe.

Erectile Dysfunction

Forget the term impotence! It's time to start talking about erectile dysfunction, abbreviated ED. It is not a simple change of vocabulary; it is above all a change in mentality and point of view. When we talk about impotence, we imagine a burdened man, a victim of a helplessly limp penis, incapable of the slightest penetration and for whom no treatment exists.

When the FDA approved Viagra in 1998, it was truly revolutionary. Doctors finally had an effective and easy-to-use drug to re-establish erectile potency. As we'll come to see, there's not just the famous Viagra but many other ways to re-establish male sexual ability. This is such a significant topic that a whole chapter is dedicated to it (see pages 122–138).

Koro

Does 黄帝内经 mean anything to you? Unless you're an accomplished sinophile, you probably can't read that text. In the Latin alphabet, these ideograms can be phonetically written as *Huangdi Nei Jing*, or the *Inner Canon of the Yellow Emperor*. It's a medical book written around five centuries ago. In the *Huangdi Nei Jing*, we find the fundamentals of traditional Chinese medicine (often abbreviated TCM), and a little something else. It's a curiosity related to the penis that is of interest to us — the description of a particular condition, called *koro*. In ideograms it is written: 缩阳 (literally: shrinking penis).

Men affected by *koro* are convinced that their penis is shrinking and will gradually disappear, as it is pulled inside their body by a force out of their control. The cause is generally reported to be either an evil spirit or poisoned food. Cases of *koro* (a Malaysian word associated with the action of a turtle pulling its head back into its shell) have been reported

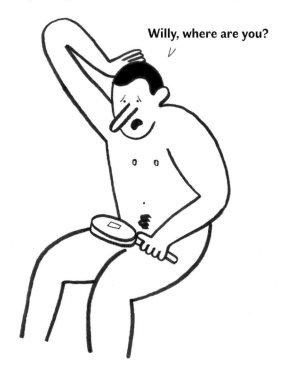

throughout Asia, including in China, Japan, Malaysia, Thailand and India. These cases can be isolated, such as when a man with a history of good health suddenly becomes alarmed to see his penis shrink. However, true epidemics have occurred, which affect thousands of people.

One *koro* epidemic took place in 1967 in Singapore and was reported in the *Singapore Medical Journal* in August that same year. The men involved were convinced that they were being poisoned by eating the meat of pigs with swine flu, and that the poisoning was demonstrated by the shrinkage or disappearance of their penis. The article describes a massive influx of men of all ages at hospitals or local doctors.

To prevent their penis from disappearing, the subjects found ingenious ways of holding on to them. Some of them taped their penis to their lower abdomen, while others tied a string to their penis and held onto it or tied the other end to a stone. More surprising still, doctors saw men who had securely attached a hair clip to their foreskin. There was even a case of a man who had inserted a skewer through his foreskin and was holding onto the skewer to try to keep his penis in place.

Koro is treated with antianxiety medications such as clorazepate, sold under the brand name Tranxene. Doctors may also prescribe antipsychotics for the most severe cases.

Peyronie's Disease

I once had a patient I knew well, who would come in for a consultation from time to time for minor health problems. One day, he seemed awkward as he sat across from me. When I asked him why he had come it, he simply said, "It's bent..." After a few questions, I made a diagnosis. This man had Peyronie's disease.

In 1743, François Gigot de La Peyronie, King Louis XV's first surgeon, described this disease that causes penile deformation, and the disease was subsequently named after him.

Peyronie's disease mostly affects men in their 50s and is relatively common, since it is estimated that 1 in 20 to 1 in 10 men suffer from it at some point in their life. The disease progresses in three stages.

1. Pain, sometimes intense pain, is felt in the penis during erection. It can be accompanied with difficulty in achieving a healthy erection. The pain is caused by inflammation of the tunica albuginea, which envelops the corpora cavernosa.

2. A few weeks or months later, the erect penis progressively curves ("It's bent"). This deformation relates to the growth of fibrous plaques in the tunica albuginea. The curvature is generally concave (i.e., upward), so much so that the glans penis points upward. The curvature is pronounced and may hinder or even prevent penetration. It progresses slowly.

3. Later, the pain subsides or even disappears, and the curvature levels off. In the best cases, the curvature gets better over the following years. In the worst cases, the curvature persists and getting an erection becomes nearly impossible.

The cause (or causes) of Peyronie's disease is unknown. It's possible that genetic factors play a role or that repetitive microtraumas are responsible. This condition is often linked to Dupuytren's contracture (which is a progressive deformity of the hand that causes one or more fingers to stay stuck in a bent position).

During an examination, the doctor will detect fibrous plaques when palpating the penis. Diagnosis is confirmed by photos of the erect penis. Here, the widespread use of smartphones has helped urologists do their work.

Until recently, treatment for Peyronie's disease was disappointing. Many products were tested, blindly, given the ignorance of the true cause of this condition. For a long time, urologists prescribed vitamin E, colchicine (the standard treatment for gout) and corticosteroids, among others, but these products have not shown many signs of improvement. The only treatment that has helped reduce the curvature is a last-resort surgery, which involves removing the fibrous plaques, but this operation is not without risk. Furthermore, the patient usually ends up with a significantly shorter penis. Surgery can also injury nerve endings, which leads to numbness of the glans and anorgasmia (i.e., inability to achieve orgasm). There is also a risk of permanent erectile dysfunction that can only be treated secondarily, with a penile implant.

I have on my shelf a medical dictionary that dates from 1895. In this large book, the authors dedicate an article to Peyronie's disease, which they called "Nodes of the Corpora Cavernosa." They describe that the nodes of the corpora cavernosa are indolent (i.e., not painful) and only cause discomfort during an erection, when the shaft bends toward the same side as the nodes. They then report that the "dangerous operation" aims to remove the nodes from the corpora cavernosa. They list the other remedies as lead iodide ointments and lotions with iodine tinctures, which they say at least improve the patient's morale.

In 2010, the FDA approved a drug for treating Peyronie's disease (it is also used to treat Dupuytren's contracture). This drug is a collagenase. It directly attacks the fibrous plaques responsible for the disease. It is administered by injections directly into the plaques. The prescribing physician then use pressure and traction on the weakened plates to straighten the penis. Collagenase is sold under the brand name Xiaflex. It is a specialized medication and is not without risks. It is approved to treat adult men with Peyronie's disease with palpable plaque and a curvature deformity of at least 30 degrees. It has been shown to reduce the curvature by 15 to 20 degrees.

Megaphallus: When the Penis Is Too Big

The motto for penises could be "the bigger, the better," since large penis size is valued in our society. However, a man with a megaphallus (also called megapenis) may not agree. He faces various difficulties. For example, his sexual partner may back away upon seeing his penis. Engaging in certain sports, like swimming, is also challenging because the silhouette of the bathing suit will prompt the curiosity of the other pool-goers. Even the simple act of wearing fitted pants is nearly impossible.

No treatment was available, and those affected simply had to deal with it. That was the situation until American urologist and surgeon Dr. Rafael Carrion, at the University of South Florida, achieved a world first: a surgical penile reduction. The procedure was performed in Tampa and was reported in the October 2014 issue of the *Journal of Sexual Medicine*.

Dr. Carrion was surprised when the patient, a 17-year-old adolescent, came in for a consultation to ask him for a penile reduction — patients generally came in asking for an inch or two or more, not less. However,

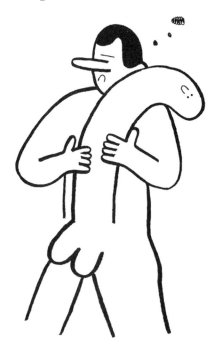

after the examination, he understood the extent of the young man's problem. His penis measured 7 inches (18 cm) when flaccid and had a circumference of 9.8 inches (25 cm). (In case you don't remember how to calculate the diameter from the circumference, you simply divide it by pi, which is 3.14.) A quick calculation shows that the diameter of the young man's penis was around 3.12 inches (8 cm), which is not common. In an interview, Dr. Carrion compared the penis to a large eggplant.

Since there was no existing operational protocol, the surgeon had to innovate. Here's a brief summary of the operation: The surgeon first made a circular incision at the base of the glans penis. He then folded the skin down, uncovering the penis. Next, he reduced the size of each corpus cavernosum.

The surgeon performed each step with great precision to avoid injuring the nerves and urethra. After two days, the patient left the clinic satisfied.

Bites

Odaxelagnia is the act of biting yourself or your partner for sexual pleasure. Biting can involve any body part, including the penis. A bite on the penis may be arousing for some, but it's much less pleasurable if the jaws close a little too tightly or if a piece of flesh is bitten right off.

From time to time, there are reports of a male victim of biting. In some cases, the incidents are a final defense against rape, but there are also cases when a betrayed spouse seeks vengeance by injuring their partner's penis

Treatment involves cleaning and suturing the wound. Antibiotics may be necessary for deep wounds. Human bites often become infected due to the presence of microbes in the mouth, such as *Eikenella corrodens*.

These wounds can heal poorly, leaving retractable and fibrotic scars, which can cause penile curvature during erection.

In case of amputation by bite, the only treatment is reimplantation. This topic is discussed in the chapter on transplants (see pages 167–173).

Edemas

Years ago, I saw a penis affected by something unusual. The patient was on sick leave and took advantage of his free time by repeatedly having sex with his partner. This led to swelling of the skin around his penis, also known as penile edema. This swelling was pronounced and practically doubled the size of his penis. I reassured the man and explained to him that no treatment was necessary; he just had to stop his sexual activity for a few days, and everything would go back to normal.

Paraphimosis

Paraphimosis is a complication of phimosis, when the foreskin that retracted behind the glans penis can't be put back in place and therefore acts as a tourniquet, causing swelling. Treatment is urgent and the first-line treatments are fairly modest remedies. Firstly, a cloth is soaked in cold water and wrapped around the penis to help bring down the swelling enough to pull the foreskin back in place. If that doesn't work, the doctor can use an anesthetic cream to numb the foreskin before attempting a reduction (a medical term that means returning a body part to its normal position). Surgery is sometimes a necessary last resort — either plastic surgery to increase the size of the foreskin (see the phimosis section on pages 102–103) or circumcision, which is the removal of foreskin (see pages 156–166).

Penis Captivus

In dogs, once the penis enters the vagina, the female encloses it in contracting muscles. This contraction, the male dog's relatively large penis and the fact that the male cannot remove his penis until he ejaculates, combine to create an effect often termed "locking" when dogs mate. This phenomenon is well known, and so is the cure: wait for the dogs to unlock themselves. There is no point in throwing water at the couple; it's useless.

Penis captivus is essentially this same "locking" phenomenon, but between people. Here is how the situation may present: A doctor is urgently called to assist a couple in full mating position, with the man's penis stuck in the woman's vagina. The course of action is not taught in school, what's to be done?

I happen to have a giant tome that's a medical dictionary that seems to have an answer for everything. It explains that you simply need to spread the woman's legs as far apart as possible, insert two fingers in her anus and then gradually pull the couple apart.

Thankfully, I have never been confronted with penis captivus, although I suppose it would make a great story to tell at conferences. Doctors like to publish articles outlining their unusual cases, but I could find only one article on penis captivus in the many medical journals I've explored. It was published in 1884 in the *Philadelphia Medical News* and written by Dr. William Osler, a famous Canadian doctor of the late 19th century. Unfortunately, it turned out this story was a hoax. However, I did find a video online of a case of penis captivus that happened in Africa. An adulterous couple who were stuck called for help, and a witness captured the scene with their smartphone.

Phimosis

In phimosis, the end of the foreskin (sometimes called the preputial ring) is too tight, which means the glans penis cannot be totally uncovered. Almost all infants have phimosis. It is very common and not considered a pathology. This particularity becomes less and less frequent as the child grows, and at three years old, the unhooding is possible in two-thirds of males. In adulthood, almost all men can unhood their glans, but some conditions (such as local infections, traumas by repetitive or too forceful unhooding, a skin disease called lichen) can tighten the foreskin and lead to a type of phimosis called acquired phimosis.

In adulthood, phimosis can be problematic for three reasons.

1. It can hinder erections or cause pain during an erection.
2. The glans and foreskin can become infected, leading to the accumulation of foul-smelling smegma. Balanitis is an infection of the glans, posthitis is an infection of the foreskin and balanoposthitis is an infection that affects both.
3. It can cause paraphimosis, which is when the foreskin has pulled by force to unhood the glans and then cannot be pulled back to its initial position. It has become blocked and then firmly tightens around the base of the glans, forming a tourniquet. This condition is discussed in detail in the paraphimosis section (see page 100).

Until recently, doctors recommended that the parents of young boys frequently pull back their foreskin while, for example, taking advantage of the relaxing effects of a bath. The drawbacks of these manipulations intended to loosen the foreskin are that they are painful and provide no health benefit.

The current recommendations are to not do anything, except in the case of a phimosis that is truly too tight. In that case, a corticosteroid cream can be used. If the cream is applied in the morning and at night for two weeks, the foreskin will become supple enough to remedy the phimosis. If that doesn't work, surgery will be necessary. It can consists of plastic surgery to enlarge the foreskin (preputioplasty) or circumcision (posthectomy).

Fish in the Penis

Candiru are a small, long fish that live in the Amazon and have a tendency of entering other fish through their gills to nibble on them from the inside, hence its nickname, the vampire fish. Candiru sometimes confuse the urinary meatus of a swimmer with a gill opening and become trapped inside the urethra. Luckily, this type of mishap is very rare. The most recent case, treated by Dr. Anoar Samad, took place in October 1997. There are leeches in rivers in Vietnam that are also known to swim "upstream" in this manner.

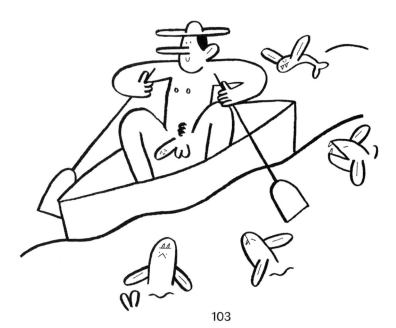

Priapism

Priapism is defined as the involuntary persistence of a complete or partial erection for more than four hours after orgasm or outside of any sexual stimulation. The term priapism comes from Priapus, the Greek god of fertility, who is depicted with an enormous penis in a constant state of erection. Urologists distinguish between ischemic priapism, also known as "low flow," which are by far the most common, and non-ischemic priapism, also called "high flow."

Ischemic Priapism

This type of priapism is an emergency. Permanent erectile dysfunction can set in within a few hours. Common causes include:

- sickle cell anemia, which causes malformation of red blood cells and is common among Africa-Americans
- intracavernous injections of alprostadil or, in particular, papaverine, which are intended to treat erectile dysfunction
- Toxins such as alcohol, cocaine and cannabis
- Certain medications, such as anticoagulants, antihypertensives, antidepressants and medications to treat benign prostatic hyperplasia

Medications to treat erectile dysfunction, like Viagra or Cialis, rarely cause priapism when the correct dosage is used, but they can cause it if they are combined with certain intracavernous injections.

A patient with priapism has a rigid and painful erection that lasts several hours. The first-line treatment to end the erection is ice wraps. If that doesn't work, the doctor will need to drain the blood from the corpora cavernosa and then inject an alpha-adrenergic stimulating agent. (This stimulant has the opposite effect of alprostadil, which is injected into the corpora cavernosa to treat erectile dysfunction.) When the stimulant is effective, the injection will stop the erection (the technical term is "detumescence"). If it fails, the surgeon must quickly turn to surgical treatment to drain the corpora cavernosa.

The simplest technique involves applying a local anesthesic and making small punctures along the glans penis toward the end of the corpora cavernosa. These holes create passages (the medical term is shunts) between the corpora cavernosa and the corpus spongiosum, which includes the glans. These shunts will allow the blood trapped in the corpora cavernosa to pass to the corpus spongiosum and the sought-after detumescence occurs. This technique carries the risk of permanent erectile dysfunction, which can generally only be treated with a penile implant. The pointed instrument used to create the punctures is hollow and has a small opening that allows the surgeon to remove a "core" by pressing it into the organ and then pulling it out. In this case, the instrument is pushed lengthwise into the glans so that it it perforates each corpus cavernosum. The core is thus a piece of corpus cavernosum, creating the shunt.

Non-ischemic Priapism

This type of priapism is secondary to a penile trauma that creates a connection between a cavernous artery and the venous system, which is called an arteriovenous fistula. The fistula causes a rush of blood and a partial erection (the technical term is tumescence).

Contrary to an ischemic priapism, this type causes some discomfort but is not terribly painful and can disappear spontaneously. Non-ischemic priapism carries less risk to the corpora cavernosa and does not require urgent treatment (surgically closing the fistula).

Allergic Reaction to Latex Condoms

Condoms are extremely useful, but they can sometimes cause problems. Most are made from latex, which is a natural substance produced from rubber trees. However, natural does not mean harmless!

Latex allergy affects 1 to 2 percent of the population and is more common in people who work at a job that involves repeatedly coming into contact with the substance, particularly health-care professionals.

Allergy to latex condoms causes local reactions in men: redness, itching and even hives (itchy red welts that form a rash on the skin). Even more rarely, this allergy can cause more troublesome systemic reactions, from difficulty breathing and general malaise to angioedema (a swelling in the deeper layers of the skin that often accompanies hives). Any time an allergic reaction involves difficulty breathing it is considered a life-threatening emergency. In females, a latex allergy causes genital irritation but can lead to serious full-body reactions. The allergy is confirmed via a skin test.

Shots don't produce useful results for this type of allergy. Sufferers simply need to avoid latex condoms. Luckily, there are non-latex condoms on the market. Most major brands sell them: LifeStyle (Skyn), Durex (Real Feel) and Trojan (BareSkin).

Frenulum Tear

One of the most memorable stories from my practice involves a frenulum tear.

During a night shift, a woman called wanting a house call as soon as possible. I received no details. I arrived at the indicated location and found a naked man seated at the edge of a bed and holding a blood-stained towel around his penis. He was panicked, of course, and his partner was no better. All I had to do was convince the man to loosen his grip on the towel to confirm what I suspected: a frenulum tear.

Remember the drawings from the penis anatomy chapter? Figure 3 (page 17) shows the parts of the glans penis, including the frenulum (4). It is a fold of skin from the glans to the foreskin. Normally, the frenulum is long enough to completely cover the glans during sex. If it is too short, it can tug a bit during the back-and-forth movements and eventually tear. This tear typically occurs during the first times a man has sex, so it often happens during adolescents, but it can also happen later in life, particularly during energetic sex. The risk is also increased when the partner is not adequately lubricated.

The frenulum has a very small, strong artery, aptly named the frenular artery. The frenulum bleeds, often profusely, when it tears. The bleeding is invariably accompanied by intense local pain.

Treatment is simple: After reassuring the injured man (and his partner!), you need to apply compression to the area with a cloth, just like the man on my shift did. Bleeding generally stops after a maximum of about 20 minutes. Once it stops, the patient should clean the area with soap and water. It is recommended to abstain from sex for two to three weeks. However, that simple treatment does not suffice, the tear must be checked to ensure that a retractile adhesion doesn't form, which would hinder future erections, and that there isn't a partial tear.

If there is an adhesion or partial tear, the patient requires a simple surgical procedure. It involves plastic surgery, which is done under local anesthesia by a urologist. Here as well, the patient must abstain from sex for three to four weeks, which is the only precaution required following this routine operation. The surgery elongates the frenulum, so once healed, the patient can resume a normal sex life without the frenulum tearing again.

Urethritis

As we saw in the chapter on penis anatomy, the urethra is a tube through which sperm and urine pass. This tube can get infected by bacteria, particularly sexually transmitted bacteria. These infections are referred to as urethritis.

While many readers may have heard of the infamous feeling of "pissing razor blades" cased by the gonococcus bacterium (gonorrhea), most cases of urethritis are caused by a baterium called *Chlamydia trachomatis*.

About one week after the infecting sex, the small bacteria cause a burning sensation during urination and a cloudy discharge. *Chlamydia trachomatis* infections have subtle symptoms that can easily go unnoticed, especially in women. This is very troublesome, since this microbe can cause infertility if it affects the fallopian tubes. *Chlamydia trachomatis* is luckily easy to get rid of with antibiotics. Most often, the doctor will prescribe a single dose of azithromycin.

Other bacteria can also lead to urethritis, including mycoplasmas, which cause problems similar to those caused by *Chlamydia trachomatis*. Treatment consists of administering macrolide antibiotics.

Gonococcus has become quite rare but unfortunately has not disappeared. A gonococcus infection differs from a *Chlamydia trachomatis* infection, and symptoms are generally more pronounced. They include:

- The infection appears more quickly (two to four days after the infecting sex).
- It causes a more intense burning sensation (often described by patients as a sensation of "pissing razor blades").
- It produces a cloudy discharge, even white or purulent, from the urethra.

Treatment also relies on antibiotics, but things do not always go smoothly, as gonococcus infections are increasingly resistant to common antibiotics. Furthermore, the bacteria often cause severe complications, particularly orchitis (infection of the testicles) and prostatitis.

To lighten the mood a bit, as this chapter is quite technical in parts, permit me to share three stories from my practice.

The first memory involves a man who spent some time at a hotel and with a partner who was not his spouse. He contracted urethritis caused by *Mycoplasma genitalium*. He came in for a consultation because of a burning sensation during urination and discharge from his urethra. Once I made the diagnosis, I prescribed the appropriate treatment and asked him to inform his wife so she could also be treated. To his credit, he did come clean. When the woman came in for a consultation, she showed me a receipt from her husband's jacket pocket proving that he had stayed at the hotel in question. She was not very surprised to be needing to visit my office for a checkup.

The second memory involves a man who took a business trip abroad. He came back with a magnificent case of gonococcal urethritis, which he contracted from vaginal sex with a sex worker. As with the last patient, I asked him to tell his wife, which he did not do, just as he refused to take a test to look for a possible co-infection with HIV (AIDS virus). I offered to tell his wife myself, which he also refused. The situation troubled me greatly, but I was bound by doctor-patient confidentiality. I later had the chance to examine his wife when she came for her regular checkup. I was relieved to see she was not suffering from any disorders, and I, of course, never informed her about her husband's health issues. It's not always easy being a doctor.

My third memory concerns a man whose wife did not want to perform fellatio. He eventually decided to go to a professional. The sex worker in question had agreed to bring my patient some happiness — without a condom. Two days later, a pus-filled discharge indicated gonococcal urethritis. This proves, if proof were needed, that the bacteria do not need vaginal intercourse to spread; it is enough that the woman gave oral sex to an infected person some time before my patient. But that's not all! My patient, burned by the experience, signed up for a well-known dating site, thinking that he could escape any diseases transmitted by sex workers. A few days later, he met up with a married woman who gave him oral sex in a parked car. Sometimes it's interesting to be a doctor. It can feel like a soap opera! I even knew the make of the car, but I'll keep that to myself. Unfortunately for my patient, the same thing happened! Well, not quite, since this time it was urethritis caused by *Chlamydia trachomatis*. Consultation, testing and antibiotic treatment followed. But wait, there's more. Thanks to the same website, our man met someone new. It was a divorced woman this time. Just like before, his new lover performed with no fuss in the car, of course with no latex in sight. The analysis of my patient's urethral discharge that followed a week later showed that despite the severe burning sensation during urination and the whitish urethral discharge suggesting gonococcus, it was also a chlamydia infection. After that, I lost touch with him.

The Penis Takeoff

It should be noted that the "takeoff" we are referring to here is the penis disappearing, not air travel — there aren't any penises bumping into clouds or perched in a tree. The disappearances, or robberies, in question occurred in Africa, and while they may have been fictitious, they had serious consequences and lead to violent deaths.

It all started in early August 1996 in Cameroon. A rumor surfaced, accusing the Hausa people of making the genitals of Cameroonians disappear. The Hausa live in Nigeria and are known for making traditional medicines that they sell throughout several African countries. The process of the so-called robbery was very simple: It was enough for a Hausa to shake the hand of a local man for him to feel a deep cold in his lower abdomen, causing his organ to retract and sometimes even disappear. Dozens of "victims" began searching for these sorcerers in order to lynch them.

When police responded, they asked the victims of the thefts to undress for verification. Everything was, of course, in order. Despite that, as days went by, the rumor grew. A report by the Agence France-Presse described men walking around with their hands deep in their pockets, refusing to shake hands.

The method varied. Sometimes, the sorcerer would only need to tap the victim on the shoulder for his penis to recoil. The punishment also varied: Some "sorcerers" were beaten to death with a stick or an iron bar, while others were immobilized by a crowd, and then tires were thrown over their bodies and sprayed with gasoline, and the unfortunate victim was burned alive.

In the weeks that followed, this deadly rumor spread across Africa, making its way to Benin, Togo, the Ivory Coast, Burkina Faso, Mali, Senegal and Mauritania, claiming multiple victims, including Hausa Yoruba and Igbo people, among others. In a few weeks, the rumor caused the deaths of 300 people and injury to 1,000 others before it was finally stopped.

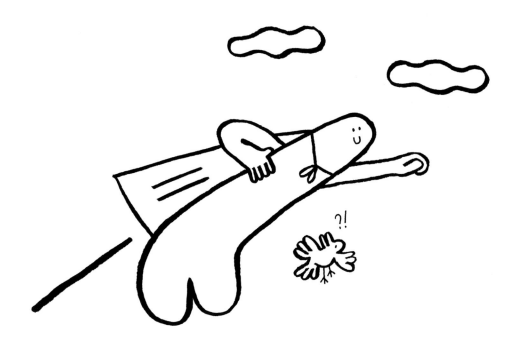

Ready To Go, But The Penis Says No: Erectile Dysfunction (ED)

"If my penis were a writer/director, it would be Woody Allen — small, neurotic, and, frankly, hit or miss."
— Matthew Norman, *Domestic Violets*

Impotence, Breakdowns, Erectile Problems, Erectile Dysfunctions and More

Most men have had at least one "breakdown," as a mechanic or sexologist might call it. It is completely normal. It's only a breakdown, and it can be fixed, often on its own. It is, however, totally different when the inability to get an erection and have a satisfying sex life is permanent.

Various studies on sexual behavior have shown that about 80 percent of men have had or have erectile problems, be it occasionally or permanently. This percentage varies by age. Among men aged 20 to 30 years, these problems are rare, while one-third of men in their early 40s and at least half of men in their 60s are affected.

One thing needs to be highlighted: erectile problems occurring in someone who up until then did not have any problems can be a warning sign. It can be related to diffuse coronary artery disease, and these men should be tested to look for risk of heart disease.

Luckily, there are many and varied solutions, as we'll see, for practically all types of erectile problems.

General Information on Causes

I own a 19th-century medical dictionary that includes a rather fanciful and old-fashioned list of causes of what we would now call erectile dysfunction (ED). This list includes myelitis, diabetes mellitus, camphor and water lily. The authors go on to list the satiey and disgust of a woman; the preoccupation of a grand idea; the fear of not performing the venereal act; the fear of syphilis; the fear of fatherhood; the energetic desire to possess a woman who, allowing herself to be caressed, then grants nothing; excessive shyness; and even magic.

While that list may seem rather muddled, it demonstrates that the main causes of ED were all, in fact, observed and documented more than 120 years ago. Today, a more detailed classification helps us distinguish whether the ED is organic, physical, psychological or caused by intoxication.

Organic ED

The causes of organic ED are far more numerous than those listed in my 19th-century reference. We can now distinguish the following causes: neurological disorders, including those caused by spinal cord damage (formerly known as myelitis); diabetes; hormonal disorders; and vascular disorders.

Neurological Causes

Neurological EDs can be caused by multiple sclerosis, Charcot joint, Parkinson's disease and similar disorders. The effects of traumatic spinal cord injuries (paraplegia or tetraplegia) are also tragic, especially because they often affect young men. Pelvic cavity surgery done to, for example, treat colon or prostate cancer, can also cause neurological damage that results in erectile problems.

Diabetes Mellitus

After several years of progression, diabetes can alter a person's arteries, particularly the small blood vessels — in other words, it can cause microangiopathies. These lesions result in a series of well-known complications: damage to the retinas, coronary arteries and kidneys and ED. Eye and heart diseases are relatively well monitored in diabetics and can be treated, but sexual disorders in these patients are too often neglected, even though they significantly lower the patient's quality of life.

Hormonal Disorders

Three hormonal dysfunctions are known to lead to erectile disorders: hypothyroidism (thyroid malfunction involving a lack of hormone secretions), hypogonadism (decrease in the secretion of testosterone) and prolactin adenoma (a benign tumor in the pituitary gland, located at the base of the brain).

Another hormonal disorder that can lead to ED is hemochromatosis. This genetic disorder results in significant absorption of iron in the digestive tract, creating an iron overload in the body. This excess of iron is absorbed by different organs, such as the liver, heart and testicles. This damage to the testicles can cause ED. This disorder most often occurs in men around the age of 40.

Vascular Disease

Atherosclerosis, the scientific name for vascular disease, is a major contributing factor to heart attacks and strokes. If a man with ED is not responding to treatments, it is good practice to confirm the state of his arteries to rule out possible atherosclerosis.

Obesity

Obesity that leads to erectile disorders is driven by two factors. First, it is often accompanied by arterial lesions caused by atherosclerosis. Second, an enzyme called aromatase that is found in excess fat turns testosterone into estrogen, which is a female hormone that can lead to ED.

ED Caused by Drugs or Alcohol

Camphor and water lily, which were once used as sedatives, can effectively decrease libido and the ability to get an erection. They are anaphrodisiacs. Potassium bromide is also an anaphrodisiac, and it was even used during World War I to decrease the sexual urges of soldiers. Here is a short story to lighten the mood:

Some years after the First World War, two former soldiers were having a conversation. One said to the other, "you know, the bromide that they put in the wine in '14, well, it's starting to take effect."

Today, substances such as camphor and potassium bromide are no longer used, but some modern and widely prescribed medications can be equally likely to cause ED.

Before continuing, I would like to emphasize a very important point. If you are treated with one of the following medications and you have ED, you should not stop taking or decrease your dose. It is essential that you consult your doctor before making any changes.

Among psychotropic medications, neuroleptic and antidepressant drugs are well-known for causing ED. Paroxetine in particular has a solid reputation as an erection killer.

In cardiology, some medications that treat high blood pressure can cause problems. They include beta-blockers (the leading one being propranolol), centrally acting antihypertensives (such as clonidine) and certain diuretics (particularly spironolactone). Statins, a class of drugs designed to lower blood cholesterol levels, are often involved in drug-induced ED. Atorvastanin in particular is closely linked with ED.

Now seems like a good time for another story from my practice...

I had just diagnosed high blood pressure in a man nearing his 70s. I prescribed him a diuretic treatment (spironolactone and altizide) and asked him to come back in three weeks to assess the drugs' effects. Eight hours later, I saw him in consultation again, this time with his wife. I quickly understood that my patient had complained that his erections had stopped and that, quite logically, he wondered if his new treatment was the cause. I explained to him that this side effect is known but rare and that I would prescribe him a different drug, one that didn't affect erections. At that moment, his wife interjected: "Yes! Another drug! With this one, erections are no longer possible!"

Medications, however, are not the only products that can cause ED. Alcohol is the leading widely used toxin that interferes with erections. Tobacco is also harmful, especially due to the arterial damage it causes. Anabolic steroids, which are hormonal substances that are popular with some bodybuilders, who use them to bulk up, often cause erectile problems with long-term use.

Psychological ED

All studies on ED show that psychological issues are by far the most frequent causes of ED. They include:

- Depressive states: a decrease in libido and the ability to get an erection are symptoms that are almost always found in depressed men. However, it is sometimes difficult to distinguish whether the ED stems from the depression itself or its treatment.
- Sexual anxiety, particularly during the first times: I have prescribed Cialis many times to young men who are nervous about a new encounter after early unsuccessful experiences with a partner who was just as inexperienced as they were.
- Weariness, burnout and overexertion can decrease desire, which often results in erectile dysfunction.

What About Magic?

In past centuries, spells involving aglet knots could be a great hardship for any man looking for love. Magical spells involving aglet knots were essentially the ancestor of the codpiece. All the wily sorcerer had to do was tie an aglet knot and render their unfortunate victim impotent. This spell was effective, provided, of course, that the person was told that a spell had been cast on him.

A famous spell book entitled *Le Grand et le Petit Albert* (the big and small Albert) includes several spells. I happen to have a 1729 edition in my home library. It teaches you how to make a woman fall in love, how to increase crops, how to increase your catch of fish, how to make amulets and how to find out the sex of a child before birth, among other spells. While ineffective, these spells at least inform us of what our ancestors were concerned about.

This famous spell book also explains how to tie the aglet knot:

Take the penis of a freshly killed wolf and stand close to the door of the person upon whom you wish to cast the spell. Call him by his name, and, as soon as he answers, tie the wolf's penis with a white lace thread. He will become so incapable of the act of Venus, he couldn't be more impotent if he were castrated.

Luckily, it was easy to break the spell:

Our ancestors assure us that the bird called the woodpecker is a remedy for the aglet knot spell if it is eaten roasted with blessed salt on an empty stomach. If one breathes in the smoke of the burnt teeth of a recently deceased man, one can likewise be delivered from the charm.

Let's return to our era (and to common sense) by summarizing the main causes of ED.

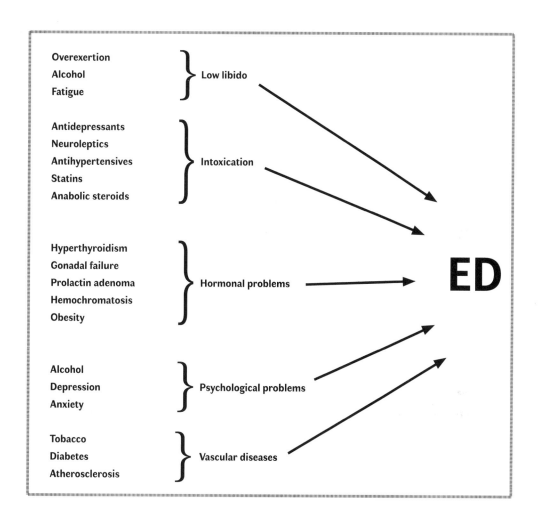

Things Are Improving! Treatments for Erectile Dysfunction

"Around the world, five times more money
is spent on breast implants and Viagra than on
Alzheimer's disease research. We can conclude
that in 30 years, there will be all kinds
of people with big boobs and magnificent erections
who can't remember what it's all for."
— Overheard at the office

Aphrodisiacs?

Aphrodisiac substances supposedly increase sexual potency. In no particular order, they include Spanish fly (an insect), hogweed (a plant), yohimbine (an extract from the bark of an African tree), rhinoceros horn, wasp larvae, swallows' nests and damiana (another plant).

Their effectiveness is highly debatable, but before Viagra, men with ED had no other options. Today, aphrodisiacs are simply an old wives' tale.

Viagra and Its Successors!

Viagra

Merriam-Webster gives the following definition for "serendipity":

The faculty or phenomenon of finding valuable or agreeable things not sought for; also, an instance of this.

Viagra is a classic example of serendipity. The pharmaceutical company Pfizer had launched a clinical study to market sildenafil citrate (the chemical name for Viagra) to treat angina. The results for that indication were not very good, but patients reported an unexpected side effect: The drug made it easy to get an erection. Research continued for this new indication, and a patent was filed in 1996. On April 1, 1998, Viagra was introduced to the market in the United States. It was an immediate success. The advent of Viagra was revolutionary because, for the first time, doctors had a drug that could effectively treat ED. The medication was introduced in Europe the following year, and it was an overnight success there too.

I had prescription requests for Viagra within weeks. Most of the time, patients would wait until the end of the consultation, while I was writing their prescription, to ask me about it. I took the time to ask a few questions and generally prescribed it to them. If I was motioning to add the drug to the bottom of the already-written prescription, the patient would often say, "No, I would prefer that it be on a different prescription." I suspected they didn't want their regular pharmacist to know about their erectile dysfunction.

Viagra is available in three doses: 25 mg, 50 mg, and 100 mg. The effective dose is typically 50 mg, but the 100 mg tablets can sometimes provide a bit of a bulk discount: It can be cheaper to buy the 100 mg pills and cut them in two than to buy the 50 mg pills.

The drug's effectiveness is visible after one hour and last from four to eight hours depending on the individual. It is important to note that sexual arousal is necessary for the drug to work. In short, Viagra helps achieve an erection by releasing an enzyme called phosphodiesterase type 5 (PDE5), which increases the amount of nitric oxide in the corpora cavernosa. (For a more detailed explanation of the medication's mode of action, see pages 32–33.)

Viagra does, however, have many contraindications. These include:

- a recent heart attack or an unstable cardiovascular state;
- the patient already taking certain other drugs, such as nitro-derivatives (which are used to treat angina and found in the street drug "poppers"), particular antibiotics, particular drugs that treat mycosis, antiviral drugs to treat HIV infection and alpha blockers (used to treat high blood pressure).

There are also numerous side effects, but these are generally minor. They include:

- facial redness (flushing, in medical terms);
- nasal congestion;
- color vision disorders;
- temporary hearing loss;
- a heart attack, particularly in the case of overdose and in men with risk factors.

Other PDE5s

Since its introduction, Viagra has made between $1 billion and S2 billion for Pfizer. This unprecedented success predictably led to imitators, and competing pharmaceutical companies introduced their own similarly acting drugs. Precautions and side effects are almost the same for these, but there are some differences.

Cialis (tadalafil) is sold by Lilly and has the significant advantage of being effective for much longer (24 to 48 hours after taking it). There are four doses: 2.5 mg, 5 mg, 10 mg and 20 mg. The 10 mg dose is generally enough. Cialis also have the advantage of not causing color vision disorders.

Stendra (avanafil) is sold by Metuchen Pharmaceuticals, has the advantage of being fast acting (15 to 30 minutes after taking it) and lasts about five hours. Three doses are available: 50 mg, 100 mg (which is typically the effective dose) and 200 mg.

Levitra (vardenafil) is sold by Bayer and has the same basic characteristics as Viagra. It is available in four doses: 2.5 mg, 5 mg, 10 mg and 20 mg.

These different medications are available by prescription only, and they can be expensive. There are foreign-based online pharmacies that offer all the PDE5s without prescription and at much lower prices than your local pharmacy. However, it is necessary to exercise extreme caution, as many of this sites sell counterfeit drugs that can contain almost anything, including toxic ingredients.

Luckily, generic brands that are much cheaper now exist for some of these drugs. Consult your doctor and pharmacist to find out which drug might best meet your needs. There are also online coupon sites that can help lower the cost of your drugs without compromising on quality — you will still purchase them from your trusted local pharmacy.

Pumps

Pumps are also called vacuums, but not quite in the sense of your vacuum cleaner. The Latin word here means "empty," and it applies to any device that helps a man achieve a passive erection by placing his penis in a transparent tube and creating a vacuum. The very first model seems to have been the "congester," which was invented by the French doctor Vincent Marie Mondat in 1826. The device was eventually forgotten about, but the idea was revived at the start of the 20th century. In 1912, a Dr. Zabludowsky began selling glass vacuums to patients in Berlin. The effect was achieved by a bike pump-like device that was connected at the bottom of a glass tube.

Both these antique devices and today's modern pumps operate in the same manner: The vacuum effect increases blood flow to the penis, causing it to swell and becomes rigid. To maintain the erection, a ring, called a tension ring, is then placed at the base of the penis. It wraps around the skin and compresses the veins, which stops the blood from flowing out of the corpus cavernosum. The size of the ring can be adjusted to ensure it does not to cause any pain.

An erection should, of course, not be maintained for too long, and it is advised to remove the ring after a maximum of 30 minutes, which is much longer than the average duration of sex (which is, according to various studies, five to six minutes excluding foreplay). Since the urethra is also compressed by the ring, sperm are not released into it at the time of orgasm. Generally, it gets propelled toward the bladder by a mechanism called retrograde ejaculation, and it then evacuates the next time the man urinates.

There are different models of pumps currently on the market. All of them have a transparent cylinder, which is necessary to see the state of the penis while it is inside. They differ by their pumping system,

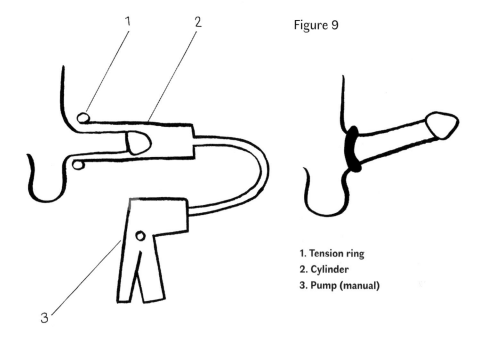

Figure 9

1. Tension ring
2. Cylinder
3. Pump (manual)

whether it is manual or electric (that latter have a small battery-pow-ered electric motor).

When buying a pump, it's important to ensure the model has an emergency air inlet button. It's a valve that allows one to quickly disen-gage the vacuum, which is very convenient in case of sudden intense pain while pumping.

The drawing above shows how to use a pump.

Using a pump is very simple, and it is easy to learn how to do it. The device is equipped with a ring at its base. The cylinder's opening must first be lubricated, and then it is held against the lower abdo-men, which needs to be shaved to prevent air from leaking out. Then, the air is pumped out. Once an erection is achieved, by increasing the blood flow, the ring is slipped onto the base of the penis and the device is removed.

A pump has two main advantages and two main disadvantages.

First advantage: it does not cost much to operate, as it can be used for a long time without requiring any maintenance. The ring may need to be changed after several years if it shows signs of wear and tear. It's a good idea to shop around. The pumps sold at sex shops are often just as effective as those sold at pharmacies but are a fraction of the cost. It's also a good idea to get a few spare rings.

Second advantage: since it produces a passive erection, a pump can be effective even if the erector nerves are injured, which can happen as a result of prostate cancer surgery.

The first inconvenience is its "lack of romance." A pump is best for couples who are understanding and can openly accept each other's weaknesses.

Another inconvenience was noted by some partners of men who use a pump: The penis is colder than one with a naturally achieved erection. That makes sense, since the blood is blocked by the ring and is no longer circulating normally.

I have twice prescribed a pump to a patient. One of the couples ultimately decided against using it, and I continued to follow the other "equipped" couple for years. Both assured me that they were quite satisfied.

Intracavernous Injections

As the term indicates, intracavernous injections are administered directly into the corpora cavernosa. More precisely, in only one of the two corpora cavernosa, since these two chambers are connected.

The first cavernous injections were administered in the early 1980s by the French doctor Ronald Virag, and the drug used at that time was papaverine. Other substances were later tried, and alprostadil is now used almost exclusively. This drug is effective and has few side effects, and, unlike papaverine, it has a low risk of priapism.

Alprostadil is sold under the brand names Caverject and Edex. Caverject is available in 20 mcg and 40 mcg doses, and Caverject Impulse is available in 10 mcg and 20 mcg dosages. Edex is available in 10 mcg, 20 mcg and 40 mcg doses. (In Canada, only the 20 mcg dosage of Caverject is available.) All forms need to be reconstituted before they can be administered. Caverject is sold in a vial, and the necessary diluent, syringes and needles must be procured separately. Caverject Impulse and Edex are sold in packs that contain all of the necessary supplies to reconstitute and inject the drug. The prescribing doctor will administer the first injection to demonstrate how to do it properly. After that, patients administer the injections themselves. It is very important to prick the side of the penis perpendicular to the skin, After disinfecting the area, the needle should be deep enough to inject the drug directly into one of the corpus cavernosum, not under the skin. Once the patient administers the injection, he must press down on the area with the pad used to disinfect the skin for two minutes to prevent a hematoma from forming.

The needle is very fine, and the injection is practically painless. The erection, achieved in about 10 minutes, is purely mechanical and does not require any sexual arousal. It generally lasts for the duration of sex. The patient should know that this erection can persist after ejaculation. These drugs are virtually 100 percent effective.

Intracavernous injections have the advantage of being effective even when the erector nerves is damaged, which can occur, which is a potential side effect of prostate cancer surgery.

Tolerance is high, and injections are only contraindicated if the patient suffers from sickle cell anemia (which is a generic disease that affects the red blood cells and is prevalent among African-Americans), as this increases the risk of priapism.

Some health insurance companies do provide at least partial coverage for these drugs. Check with your provider, particularly if you are affected by any of the following:

- paraplegia or tetraplegia;
- multiple sclerosis;
- diabetic neuropathy;
- pelvic trauma complicated by urinary disorders;
- prostatectomy;
- cystectomy (removal of the bladder);
- colorectal surgery;
- pelvic radiation therapy;
- priapism.

MUSE

MUSE is the acronym for Medicated Urethral System for Erection. It is a plastic device that allows a patient to introduce into the urethra a small suppository (0.05 inches / 1.4 mm in diameter) that contains the active drug alprostadil. It is available in four doses: 0.125 mg, 0.25 mg, 0.5 mg and 1 mg. MUSE consists of a plastic body fitted with a button and a very slim stem that allows the medication to be inserted directly into the urethra. This stem is sterile and protected by a cap. As with intravcavernous injections, MUSE delivers alprostadil, so it is contraindicated for patients with sickle cell anemia.

It is simple to use:

- Urinate and then wash the hands.
- Remove the cap; once the cap is removed, never touch the stem.
- Pull the penis upward with one hand.
- Hold MUSE in the other hand and gently insert the stem into the urethra.
- Press the button all the way down with your index finger.
- Gently remove the device.
- Roll the penis between both hands for about 10 seconds to distribute the drug.
- It is recommended to walk for a few minutes to stimulate circulation.
- An erection is usually achieved after 5 to 10 minutes and lasts 30 to 60 minutes. It is possible for it to persist after ejaculation.

Side effects are rare and mostly local. They include:

- a burning sensation in the urethra,
- bleeding, particularly in men being treated with anticoagulants;
- general disorders such as dizziness and low blood pressure, which are even rarer.

While intracavernous injections tout a success rate of nearly 100 percent, MUSE is not as effective, despite the fact that it contains the same active drug. This is likely because to reach the corpora cavernosa, the alprostadil delivered by MUSE must travel through the urethra and then spread to the corpus spongiosum, and the rate of diffusion varies depending on the individual.

Implants

Implants are recommended only as a last resort, when all other solutions have failed or are not suitable for the patient. Implants are inserted in the corpora cavernosa, and they can be either semirigid or inflatable.

Semirigid implants are made of silicone and have a metal core. They are also malleable and can be directed upward, for an erection, or downward. They have the advantage of being simple to use, but they are not always discreet.

For years, I followed a patient who had this kind of prothesis. The first time that I saw him in his underwear, lying down on the exam table, I noticed right away that he had a bulge in his underwear. I must have looked surprised, as he reassured me by saying that he had a prothesis. It suited him just fine, and he was the life of the party at his retirement home.

Figure 10

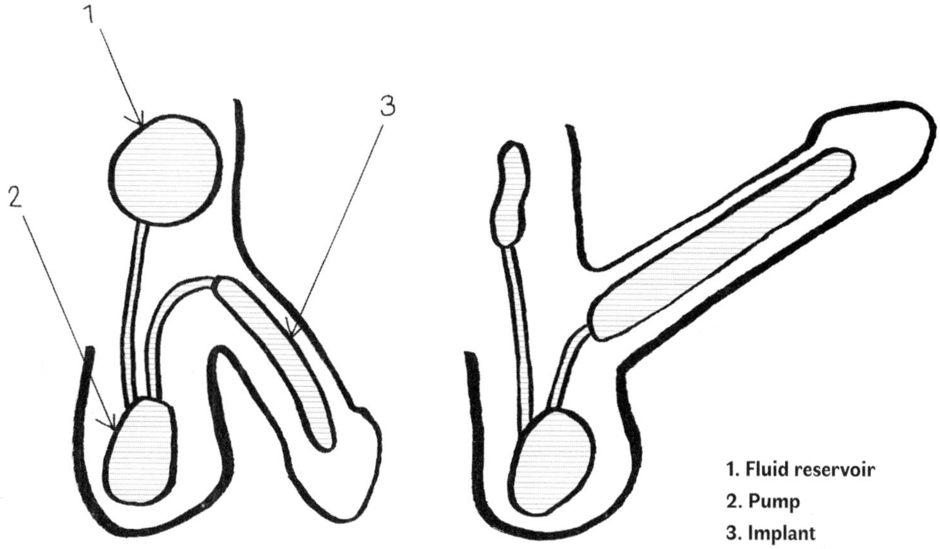

1. Fluid reservoir
2. Pump
3. Implant

Inflatable implants are much more sophisticated. As shown in figure 10, they are made a pair of implants (3), which are inserted into the two corpora cavernosa, a fluid reservoir (1), which is placed in the lower abdominal area, and a pump (2), which is placed in the scrotum, like a third testicle.

The procedure to implant the device takes a little more than an hour. Complications are possible but rare. They include:

- infection, which sometimes requires removing the implant;
- hematomas;
- mechanical failure, which can require another surgery;
- the glans penis can erode over time, and in extreme cases the implant eventually can poke through the skin.

Sex is possible after a postoperative recovery period of 6 to 8 weeks to allow the patient to heal.

There is a bit of learning curve when it comes to using the implant. The recipient pumps the fluid (saline) from the reservoir, sending it into the implants in the corpora cavernosa. These become rigid and remain that way as long as necessary. Once sex is over, the person just needs to press on the valve located on the pump to return things to a resting state.

Most people with a prosthesis, and their partners, are satisfied. Dissatisfaction usually comes from the fact that the glans penis remains soft and doesn't have a natural appearance.

Some health insurance providers cover implants. Check with yours to confirm.

Products Available in the Near Future

Viagra Condoms?

Recently, condoms sold under the brand name Blue Diamond have hit the European market. They claim not to cause an erection but to increase the penile stiffness of those who use them. These condoms contain Zanifil gel in their "teat" (or reservoir). The gel is thereby in close contact with the glans penis and absorbed by it. Condoms that could be available without a prescription and help compensate for an erection that's a little, say, hesitant is very interesting! Let's take a closer look.

Trinitrin, which is well-known by cardiologists, who have used it for decades to treat heart attacks, is simply nitroglycerine, a famously explosive substance. It works by dilating blood vessels, which is how it stops an angina attack. Trinitrin acts through nitric oxide (NO), which is an integral part of the erection mechanism. Another name for trinitrin is glyceryl trinitrate, which is the active agent in Zanifil.

In short, Blue Diamond condoms act by the penetration of NO, from the trinitrin gel, through the surface of the glans. This use seems logical, since the drug is a vasodilator; therefore, it is likely to increase blood flow to the corpora cavernosa, the executors of erections.

While these condoms may be getting a reputation as the "Viagra" condoms, it must be emphasized that the use of any nitrate drug, including the Blue Diamond condom, is strictly contraindicated in combination with Viagra, Cialis, Stenra, Levitra and similar drugs. There is a dangerous risk of a significant drop in blood pressure.

These condoms are not yet available in the United States or Canada, but they may make an appearance soon.

New Forms of Alprostadil

Alprostadil is already available via intracavernous injections (Caverject and Edex) and urethral mini-suppository (MUSE), and creams have been researched and undergone trials in both the United States and Canada, but none is yet approved. A product called Vitaros has been available in Europe for a few years. It is dispensed in a mini-syringe and inserted directly into the urinary meatus.

The next generation of alprostadil creams will likely be applied directly on the glans penis or the skin of the penis. These newer creams contain a substance called SEPA (which stands for soft enhancement of percutaneous absorption), which encourages the active drug to pass through the skin. Thanks to this substance, the alprostadil will be able to penetrate into the corpora cavernosa to increase blood flow, which leads to an erection. Topical application is far less invasive than the delivery methods currently approved. Alprostadil is rarely prescribed, but this convenient form may make it more popular.

In China, this cream has been available since October 2011 under the name Alprox-TD. The pharmaceutical company that makes it has requested authorization to sell it in the United States, Canada and Europe. Another similar product manufactured by the American company MacroChem may soon be available in the United States under the brand name Topiglan.

Shock Wave Therapy

Studies have recently been conducted, most notably at Tenon Hospital in Paris and the faculty of medicine at Sapienza University in Rome, to assess the efficacy of shock waves for the treatment of vascular ED. This treatment had already been tested to treat patients suffering from angina who were unresponsive to usual therapies, but it is still in the experimental stage. Shock wave therapy consists of sending bursts of ultrasounds to an area of the body, in this case the penis, to promote the appearance of new blood vessels (in scientific terms, it is referred to as promoting neovascularization), which improves blood flow. Current research aims to make PDE5s effective for people who are not responding to those drugs. Given the mode of action, the trials focused on people with ED associated with heavy smoking or who suffer from angina. The results, obtained by the Italian researchers and published in May 2016 in *The Journal of Urology*, are promising. However, other medical teams working on the same procedure obtained significantly worse results. These were published in *The Journal of Sexual Medicine* in March 2017.

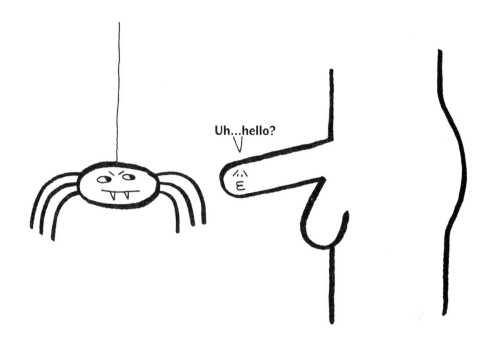

A Drug Derived from the Wandering Spider

Phoneutria nigriventer is a large venomous spider, measuring 2 inches (5 cm) long. It is commonly known as the wandering spider or armed spider and is often found in bunches of bananas. They are found in Central America and South America, particularly in Brazil, hence they are sometimes called the Brazilian wandering spider. A bite from *Phoneutria nigriventer* causes redness and an edema at the site, nausea, vomiting, general malaise and even a loss of consciousness.

Those are fairly commonplace reactions to a spider bite, but this spider's venom also causes priapism, meaning it causes a prolonged erection.

Brazilian researchers studied the venom and isolated two substances, which they called PnPP-19 and PnTx2-6. They then tested these two peptides on rats and observed that they caused erections, but without the other problems that usually occur due to the spider's bite. Better yet, the first toxin did not need to be injected; it just needed to be applied to the rats' skin to induce an erection after about 20 minutes.

The mode of action is only just starting to be understood. The venom from this spider acts through nitric oxide, the famous NO that's found in the mechanism of an erection. Results were published in *The Journal of Sexual Medicine*. In the coming years, Viagra may well have some competition!

Gene Therapy for ED

Several pharmaceutical companies are studying the possibility of gene therapy for ED. The idea is simple: A gene, known as NOS3 and present on human chromosome 7, will be isolated and injected directly into the corpora cavernosa. This gene makes it possible to produce larger quantities of NO synthase, an enzyme that enables the synthesis of NO (nitric oxide), which plays a central role in the mechanism of an erection. If those studies are successful, the big advantage of this treatment would be that only one injection every year would be required.

Incisions and Other Injuries: The Mistreated Penis

*"My penis is like a burn victim after I orgasm.
Don't get near it. It hurts. Leave it be."*
— Adam Carolla

When it comes to body modification, the human imagination is endless, and there are many ways to mistreat the penis to realize many types of objectives. Some are relatively mild, like tattoos, but others are closer to psychiatric issues rather than urological ones.

Penis Splitting

This major mutilation, which is almost certainly in the domain of psychopathology rather than urology — involves separating the two corpora cavernosa all the way to the base of the shaft. The corpus spongiosum is sacrificed, the urethra drains at the scrotum and the man must sit to urinate. The result is two semi-penises that are only capable of erection in some cases and for which ejaculation occurs at the scrotum.

Figure 11

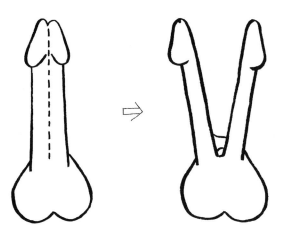

Foreign Bodies

When I was a student, I interned in a urology department at a hospital. The department head had carefully preserved in a glass cabinet the different objects that he had removed from his patients' urinary tracts over the years. When a new batch of interns arrived, the department tour included a visit to this small museum. Women have a shorter urethra, so foreign objects were generally easily found in the bladder. In men, however, they usually remained stuck in the urethra. In that famous cabinet, there were pieces of electrical wire, a fair number of hairpins, candles, bird feathers, nails, screws, pencils, pen caps, pens and many other objects.

These various findings show that urethral masturbation is not rare. In fact, there are urethral plugs and jewelry. These are thin objects made of stainless steel or plastic that are designed to be inserted into the urethra. Lovers don't even need to go to a sex shop to get them, as they can now be purchased online. I suspect my old department head is going to need to get a bigger showcase...

Medical journals have published cases involving surgeries to remove unusual object's from men's urethras. Dr. Krishanth Naidu of Canberra, Australia published in the *International Journal of Surgery Case Reports* a case involving a 70-year-old man who needed surgery to remove a fork he had inserted into his urethra for erotic purposes. One can only hope he inserted the handle rather than the tines... Meanwhile in Harbin, China, Dr. Xu Liyan removed a USB cable from a young man's urethra. Perhaps he was looking to invent urethral masturbation 2.0? Progress never stops...

Penis Cryotherapy

There are two types of cryotherapy. The first involves very local application of intense cold on the skin to freeze it and destroy any diseased tissue. This is how, for example, dermatologists treat warts.

The second type of cryotherapy is a more recent invention and involves exposing the whole body or an area of the body to an extreme cold achieved through liquid nitrogen vaporization. For whole body exposure, the treated person is placed in a cryogenic chamber for a few minutes. The temperature in the chamber is −184°F (−120°C).

Enthusiasts tout the beneficial effects with respect to inflammation and immunity.

Some doctors have tried to apply the second type of cryotherapy to the penis. It's exposed to liquid nitrogen vapor for a few moments, long enough for the skin's surface to freeze but short enough to avoid damaging the deeper layers of skin. The safe zone for this treatment is a very short window of time, which makes this therapy potentially dangerous. The desired effect is rejuvenating skin (which will peel in the days that follow and be replaced with new skin) and improving erectile capacity (through the effect the cold has on the blood vessels). There is no scientific data that demonstrates the efficacy of this treatment.

Looking for Enlightenment

Many years ago, I treated a young African woman who reported suffering from irritations in different areas of her body. She explained that these irritations could only be relieved by corticosteroid-based creams. Curiously, during our consultations, I never noticed any visible irritation. However, I trusted her and prescribed her a drug from the corticosteroid family.

It is worth noting that topical corticosteroids are divided into four groups, ranging from I to IV, according to their potency. Group I products are highly potent and are associated with many side effects. In practice, this group is reserved for conditions that cannot be otherwise treated. At the other end of the spectrum, group IV products are much less potent but are associated with very few side effects. Best practice recommends limiting prescriptions to the least potent drug possible. With that in mind, I prescribed a group IV drug to my patient.

The following day, she returned to see me and asked for a more potent drug. She had brought with her a list of group I drugs. I refused to prescribe any of these drugs to her, and I never saw her again.

In that case, I firmly believe she intended to misuse her medication. Corticosteroid creams are sometimes used by women of color to bleach their skin. Very large quantities of the creams must be used over a long period of time to achieve a visible result. This is a significant misuse of these products, and possible side effects include serious skin damage and general disorders, such as high blood pressure and diabetes.

Men also sometimes misuse corticosteroid creams to bleach their genitals, penis or scrotum. However, corticosteroid creams are not the only products misused in the manner. Other chemical products that can be used to lighten the skin include hydroquinone-based preparations. This compound is familiar to anyone who has developed their own photographs.

Genital bleaching is prevalent in Thailand, and a hospital in the Bangkok region, Lelux Hospital, has innovated the practice by offering penis bleaching using a laser. The technique is not without dangers, however, and carries a significant risk of burns and pigmented scars. The penis will suffer, as will the wallet: Five sessions costs more than $600, while the average monthly salary in Thailand is about $570.

The Lelux Hospital had already gained a certain notoriety before they began bleaching genitals with lasers. A few years earlier, they offered their female clients a service to "resculpt" their vagina by injecting fat from the abdomen into their labia majora. They promised to make the genitalia of these women plumper and more "desirable." This procedure was called 3D Vagina.

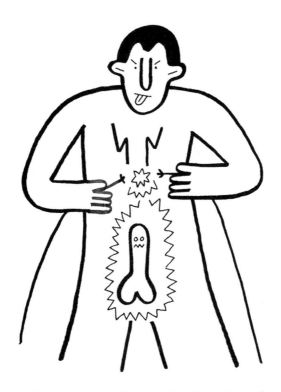

Electrocution of the Penis

Many years ago, a young man came in for a consultation for a bizarre "problem." He would give himself a thrill using a telephone magneto he had bought at a flea market. This little device was a small generator operated by a crank. It provided 10 volts of low intensity current and was once used to power telephone ringers. The young man would connect one of the two current output wires to a metal object inserted in his anus and wing the bare end of the other wire around his penis. He would then turn the crank. Far from the wonderful sensations he was looking for, he saw a series of flashing lights. He was now coming in for a consultation to ask me what had happened. I suspected there was an electrical stimulation of the retina or brain, but I was unable to provide him with a medical explanation. I encouraged him to consult a psychiatrist, concerned he might inadvertently hurt himself. He refused.

It seems that my young patient was not the only one interested in electrical stimulation. It took me less than a minute to find a similar device on the Internet. For about $50, you can procure an "Electro orgasm sex kit, cock ring, nipple clamps and anal plug toy." It would be quite versatile, since it can stimulate the penis as well as the nipples and the end of the digestive tract.

The description under the device's photo states:

- It's a fun toy for BDMS, making women more feminine and sexy.
- Use a low current and apply to the body's sensitive areas.
- Achieve the highest level of pleasure.
- This feeling is not something that everyone has tried.

Infibulation

This practice is akin to kynodesme, which will be discussed in the chapter dedicated to penis apparel (see page 178). Infibulation itself was popular in ancient Greece. It involved piercing two small holes in the foreskin and letting them heal but not close. The two permanent holes allowed a ring or a pin to pass through to close the foreskin. This pin was later called a fibula by the Romans, who also embraced it, which gives us the term we use in English today as the name of the small bone between the knee and ankle.

Infibulation didn't interfere with urination; its purpose was to prevent sexual intercourse and thus prevent the discharge of sperm. Ancient Greeks believed sperm contained a sort of "vital force" and that discharging it weakened men. Athletes were expected to remain chaste. It was also recommended that singers not ejaculate to preserve their beautiful voices. In *On the Usefulness of the Parts of the Body*, the Greek physician Galen explains that:

The vital breath is discharged from the arteries together with the seminal fluid: Therefore, it is not surprising that people who are engaged in libertinism become weak, since the purest of each of the two materials is removed from throughout the body.

Meatotomy

This body modification falls under the category of "DIY" masochism. It involves splitting the urinary meatus along the length of the glans penis. The patient is left with a bifid glans. He can still urinate standing up, but he may not always be able to control the direction of the stream. When the operation is done in a medical setting, an electric scalpel is generally used, which helps prevent profuse bleeding. If meatotomy is done by hand, the tool is usually a simple sharp blade, and the risk of bleeding is quite high.

Penectomy

A penectomy is the removal of the penis. It can be performed for medical reasons, sex reassignment, punishment or even religious reasons.

Penectomy for medical reasons is done in practice only for cancers that cannot be treated otherwise. Removal can be partial or complete. It is interesting to note that the recipient of the first penis transplant with a donor performed in the United States was a man whose penis was amputated due to cancer.

I have a medical dictionary from 1895 that outlines three ways to perform a penectomy. In the first method, a scalpel was used to make an incision and the skin of the penis was retracted. The surgeon was then to make a single cut, tie the dorsal arteries of the penis and cauterize the surface of the corpora cavernosa with a hot iron. The second method they recommend is linear crushing, which they advise is just as good as making an incision. The third and final method involves amputating the penis using a ligature made of a strong wire. They advise inserting a metal probe in the urethra and waiting for the penis to fall off.

In male-to-female sex reassignment surgery, the penis is not usually completely removed. Part of the glans can be used to create the neoclitoris, and the skin, after the corpora cavernosa and corpus spongiosum are removed, can be used to create a neovagina.

In the past, men were sometimes sentenced to having their penis removed as punishment for sexual offences or other crimes. This practice was once found in China to punish men who committed adultary. Women were punished with imprisonment. In Japan, penectomy was practiced as an alternative to capital punishment.

The Skoptsy were a Christian sect that emerged at the end 18th century in Russia. The term "Skoptsy" came from the Russian word meaning "eunuch." Members of this sect advocated castration. In females, the two breasts were removed, while men could perform the "lesser seal," which consisted of removing "only" their testicles, or the "greater seal," which was more complete since the penis was also removed. The Skoptsy believed evil stemmed from sexuality, and they hoped to achieve perfection through these mutilations. As curious as that may seem, this sect was successful and welcomed thousands of members, many hundreds of whom were castrated. It lasted into the early 20th century.

Still on the topic of religion, but in a more abstract sense, the penises of naked male statues at the Vatican have been either covered with a leaf or broken off. It appears to be the work of Pope Pius IX, and it is believed that the removed penises are kept hidden in an annex of the Vatican Museum.

Pearls

Pearls (or similar items) can be inserted under the skin of the penis and left there permanently. Once healed, you get a bumpy penis that is supposed to give your partner more pleasure.

This practice has long been observed in several parts of Asia. In Korea is it known as *chagan* balls, in Thailand, it is called *fang muk* and in the Philippines it is *bulletus*. Pearls are sometimes inserted on the penis to help prevent *koro* (the disappearance of the penis; see pages 94–95). Penis pearls are also said to be common among the yakuza, a powerful Japanese crime organization. A survey conducted in a Japanese prison revealed that 22 percent of inmates had these implants.

The practice of implanting penis pearls has recently spread worldwide, and in the United States it is known as penile marbles or love pearls.

The procedure is traditionally done in prisons, in very rudimentary hygiene conditions. A penile incision is done with a razor blade among the best-equipped operators, while others must content themselves with the lid from a can, sharpening it by rubbing it on a cement floor. The skin is then peeled back, and the pearl is inserted. Healing can take a long, time and the process is generally very painful.

Outside of prisons, pearls are implanted in hygienic conditions and made of glass, silicone, surgical steel or titanium.

In prison, the implants are made from whatever material is available: pieces of melted plastic, rounded stones, ball bearings, etc. In recent years, the trend was to use pieces of a plastic toothbrush handle. The pieces, of varying lengths — some measuring almost 1 inch (2 cm) have been found — are rounded and polished. A study carried out at Remire-Montjoly prison in Cayenne, French Guiana, revealed that among the 450 examined inmates, 243 had these "pearl" implants, with some having up to 15.

Pearl implantation is a very painful process, and infectious complications are common: local infections, which can end up as penile necrosis, and even the transmission of viruses like hepatitis and AIDS.

The risks do not end once the man is fully healed. Complications include delayed necroses and breaking condoms. The partners of these customized men may experience vaginal or anal erosions or wounds.

Piercings of All Kinds

Just like tattoos, piercings have existed for a very long time, but they were generally limited to the ears and nose. However, since the 1980s, piercings have branched out and can be done on practically any part of the body. Some are meant to be seen, like the lip, nose and ears, while others are more intimate, like the belly button or genitals.

When it comes to areas other than the ears and nose, there are two main types of jewelry: the barbell, which consists of a curved bar with a ball that screws on at each end, and the ring, which can be permanently fixed or closed by a screwed ball, which allows it to be removed. And material matters — the piercing must not oxidize and should be as hypoallergenic as possible. Surgical stainless steel is widely used, but there are also piercings made from titanium or even platinum.

Figure 12

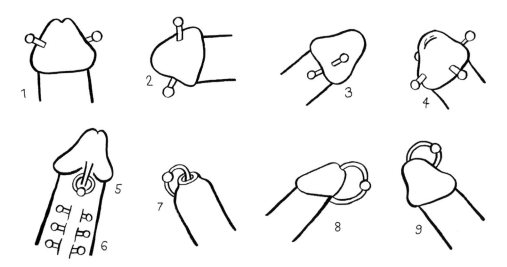

1. Ampallang 2. Apadravya 3. Dydoe 4. Magic cross 5. Frenum
6. Frenum ladder 7. Oetang 8. Prince Albert 9. Reverse Prince Albert

Getting a penis piercing is accompanied by immediate discomfort and opens one up to problems later on. At the time of the piercing, the pain can be intense, particularly in the glans, which is a very sensitive area. Bleeding can be profuse, particularly when the piercing goes through the corpora cavernosa, which are more or less blood-soaked sponges. There is also a risk of infection, and even local infections can turn into gangrene. Healing takes two to six months, depending on the individual and the placement of the piercing. Although some of these piercings are meant to increase the partner's pleasure during sex, they can also cause injuries (particularly a risk of tearing) in both the partner and the pierced individual.

These are the main types of male genital piercings.

1. Ampallang: This is a traditional piercing among the Dayak people in Borneo, where it is part of their initiation rites. It goes through the glans penis horizontally. It is recommended

that it be done on an erect penis. The *ampallang* is known to hemorrhage badly.

2. Apadravya: This is a traditional piercing in India. It is inserted not horizontally but vertically, and it goes through the glans penis and urethra.

3. Dydoe: In practice, this piercing can only be done on circumcised men. It passes through the ridge of the glans penis's base. This is the most painful type of piercing. There are single and double dydoes.

4. Magic cross: This is a combination of the *ampallang* and *apadravya*, so one piercing is horizontal and the other is vertical. It can be done in one or two sessions.

5. Frenum: This piercing generally uses a ring that passes through the frenulum of the glans penis. There is also a variant that is placed much lower on the shaft, at the base of the underside of the penis. This variant is called a lorum piercing.

6. Frenum ladder: Enthusiasts sometimes get additional frenum piercings all along the skin covering the underside of the corpus spongiosum, forming a frenum ladder.

7. Oetang: A ring passes through the foreskin, a bit like infibulation, but it remains free and is not meant to close the foreskin.

8. Prince Albert: Rumor has it that Albert of Saxe-Corbug and Gotha, husband of Queen Victoria, had this type of piercing. A ring goes through the underside of the glans penis and into the urethra.

9. Reverse Prince Albert: This is a ring that passes through the top of the glans penis.

Penile Bloodletting

The Maya civilization is known for its rich culture that included beautiful architecture and a very precise calendar. They are also known for having a bit of an appetite for human sacrifices. In addition to the massacres of prisoners and children, the king himself wouldn't hesitate to get involved during ceremonies by cutting his penis (with a blade made from obsidian) to let his blood run. This blood was collected on leaves that were then burned; the smoke was believed to go up toward the gods.

Subincision

Subincision involves opening the urethra from the urinary meatus toward the base of the penis, along a short or long length. In the most extreme cases, the urethra is opened all the way to the base of the penis. The result is a disfigured penis that is a bit flattened and resembles a vulva. The end of the urethra is in that case anastomosed (i.e., joined) with the base of the penis. A man with this extreme form of subincision must sit down to urinate, since he cannot aim. Some opt to place a tube at the opening of their urethra in order to from a standing position.

Subincision is different from bifurcation, as the two corpora cavernosa remain connected lengthwise.

Subincision is traditional among the Aboriginal tribes of central Australia, where it is considered a rite of passage into adulthood and called *mika*. It is also found in regions of Africa, South America and Polynesia.

Figure 13

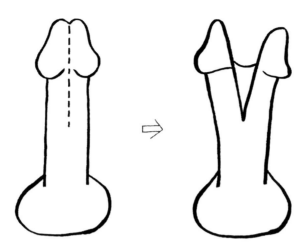

Tattoos

As tattoos have become increasingly popular, they have started to adorn all areas of the body, including the most intimate areas, such as the anus and penis. The interested reader can surely find numerous examples online.

There are generally no issues with penis tattoos, except for local pain that can be intense. Oversight and health regulations for tattoo studios have improved over the years, and infections, once common, are becoming increasingly rare.

The February 2011 issue of the *Journal of Sexual Medicine* reports a rare complication from a tattoo in an area that is of interest to us. A 21-year-old Iranian man had the terrible idea of getting a message tattooed on his penis: Good luck on your travels. The name of his lover started with an M, so he had this letter added to his glans penis for good measure. The tattooed man experienced intense local pain for the next week, and then a semi-erection popped up and stayed that way. A little worried, he consulted with doctors at Kermanshah University of Medical Sciences, who diagnosed a non-ischemic priapism that was caused by the tattoo needle perforating a cavernous artery. This perforation led to the permanent passage of arterial blood into the corpora cavernosa, hence the erection, or rather turgescence; while the penis's volume had permanently increased, it was not completely rigid. Various treatments were tried, without success. *The Journal of Sexual Medicine* concludes by stating that the patient was ultimately not that upset and decided to stop treatment and keep his permanent semi-erection.

Penile Strangulation

The term "cock ring" is self-explanatory. This sex toy, which can be made of plastic, metal, leather, rubber or silicone, is placed at the base of the penis before an erection. The cock ring works by causing strangulation of the penis.

Once erection is achieved, the ring increases pressure in the corpora cavernosa, which helps the erection become more rigid. The cock ring also encircles the corpus spongiosum, which enlarges the glans penis by increasing the blood pressure. Since the corpus spongiosum is compressed, the urethra is also crushed, so sperm cannot escape from the body. That is called a retrograde ejaculation; the sperm go into the bladder, not outside the body.

My trusty 19th-century medical dictionary contains a few sentences dedicated to penile strangulation by a constricting tie or ring. The authors explain that strangulation of the penis by foreign bodies establishes tumefaction (i.e., swelling) of all the areas situated ahead of the constricting ring. They caution that the swelling can sometimes engulf the constricting agent in edematous tissue. They provide the following list of possible constricting agents: a tie of fabric or thread, a ring, a bobeche, a bayonet mount, a faucet ferrule and the neck of a glass bottle. They also note there may be other, more exceptional cases.

When all goes well, the wearer will not have any difficulty removing the ring after ejaculation and detumescence. Unfortunately, problems do sometimes occur. The erection can persist, which can cause the ring to embed in the flesh, and the wearer will be unable to remove it. This can lead to ischemic priapism with all of the possible complications of that condition, including permanent erectile dysfunction.

Treatment consists of cutting the ring in a clinic or hospital, which can be easy to do or more difficult, depending on the situation. For example, bolt cutters are usually required to cut a metal ring, and not all emergency rooms have a pair handy...

Due to the urethra being crushed, if the ring cannot be quickly removed, a man who suffers from priapism due to a cock ring will not be able to urinate and risks going into urinary retention. Urethral crushing also makes it impossible to insert a probe, so the retention can only be treated by puncturing the bladder with a needle inserted above the pubis (called a suprapubic catheter).

Long story short, if you are tempted to try a cock ring, it is best to choose one made of a pliable material such as silicone or rubber.

Circumcision: Removal and Reconstruction of the Foreskin

The Definition of Circumcision

Circumcision is the removal of the foreskin, leaving the glans penis permanently uncovered. In practice, this removal can be partial or complete. The frenulum may also be removed or kept intact. When circumcision is carried out for medical reasons, it's called posthectomy.

Circumcision Through the Lens of a Surgeon

The official position of both the American Academy of Pediatrics (AAP) and the Centers for Disease Control and Prevention (CDC) is that current evidence indicates the health benefits of newborn male circumcision outweigh the risks. The AAP identifies the specific benefits as the prevention of:

- urinary tract infections
- acquisition of HIV,
- transmission of some sexually transmitted infections, and
- penile cancer.

In Canada, meanwhile, the Canadian Paediatric Society's position statement does not support circumcision in all cases. They recognize there may be benefits for some boys in high-risk populations, but they do not recommend the routine circumcision of every newborn male.

In my view, a surgeon should only perform a posthectomy if there is a medical reason. By this I mean:
- a very tight phimosis that leads to discomfort,
- one or more instances of paraphimosis, in order to prevent relapses, or
- recurrent infections of the glans penis (called balanitis, see pages 78–80) or of both the glans penis and the foreskin (called balanoposthitis).

However, I do not believe the decision to perform a posthectomy should ever be rushed. For example, phimosis in the first years of life is completely normal and does not require surgery in all cases. Things generally improve on their own.

In the late 19th century and early 20th century, circumcisions were performed to "cure" masturbation, and the practice was not limited to boys. Surgeons of that era didn't hesitate to surgically remove the labia minora of girls who masturbated, which is now recognized as being completely normal and necessary for sexual fulfillment. This type of mutilation is no longer practiced in most areas of the world.

A posthectomy can also be performed to prevent a religiously motivated circumcision from being done in unsanitary conditions, which

Figure 14

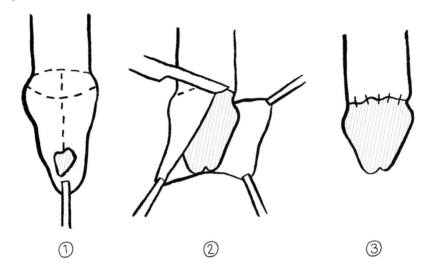

①   ②   ③

could lead to dangerous complications. Many times, I have sent a young boy to my corresponding urologist for a religious circumcision; the procedures proceeded without difficulty.

There are two types of procedures in current practice:

- A conventional circumcision
- A preputioplasty

This latter procedure is indicated for phimosis and less invasive, enlarging the preputial ring without actually removing anything.

Here is how a surgeon performs each of these two procedures.

In a conventional circumcision, the surgeon pulls the foreskin down, makes a longitudinal incision (1) followed by a circular incision, which detaches the foreskin (2) and uncovers the glans penis. The surgeon then makes a suture to connect the skin and the mucous membrane (3). There are several other types of posthectomy; some techniques require the use of a plastic ring, although that technique is mainly used on small children.

Preputioplasty, also called the Duhamel procedure, is indicated for the surgical treatment of phimosis. The surgeon first tightens the phimosis. They then retract the foreskin behind the glans, thus creating a paraphimosis, and make an incision. The surgeon then spreads the sides of the cut apart, transforming the longitudinal incision into a lateral incision, and then sutures it. The preputial ring is now significantly larger, which allows the foreskin to retract over the glans without any problems, which prevents paraphimosis.

Some complications can occur, including local edemas, prolonged bleeding, infection and impaired healing (particularly in diabetics). However, the aftercare of these two types of procedures is generally simple.

Smegma is produced by the preputial glands; once the foreskin is removed, this substance disappears.

Circumcision Through the Lens of a Hygienist

Several studies, particularly studies conducted in Kenya and Uganda, have demonstrated that circumcision reduces the risk of men being infected by AIDS by about 60 percent. This is due to the fact that circumcision removed a soft area of the mucous membrane. Since the 2000s, the UNAIDS Programme recommends circumcision in developing countries to reduce the risk of infection with HIV and reduce its spread. Several campaigns have been implemented, and hundreds of thousands of African men have been circumcised in an effort to help stop the spread of AIDS.

Circumcision Through the Lens of a Sexologist

Some believe that circumcision deprives the person of two areas that are rich in nerve endings and that play a major role in achieving pleasure: the inside surface of the foreskin and the frenulum (when it is removed, which is often the case). What's more, because of its permanent exposure to friction, it is theorized that the surface of the glans can thicken. In medical terms, it would be said to keratinize. This keratinization would make it less sensitive.

Several studies have been conducted to see if circumcised men experience less pleasure during sex, but for now they have not provided a clear answer. Some studies claim that circumcised men experience the same sensations as other men, while other studies have come to the opposite conclusion.

It does, however, seem that circumcised men suffer from fewer premature ejaculations than uncircumcised men. This also relates to the change in the surface of the glans penis, which becomes less sensitive. As for female partners, no study has reported any difference in terms of their satisfaction in relation to the presence of a foreskin or lack thereof.

Circumcision Through the Lens of Religion

I am well-versed in the field of medicine, but not at all in that of religion. This section is therefore rather brief.

Circumcision is not required by most Christian religions. The exceptions are certain Evangelical denominations and Egyptian Copts.

Among the Jewish, circumcision is practically mandatory. It is called a bris and is performed on the eighth day of life by a specially trained person called a *mohel*. In practice, the foreskin should be buried once it is removed.

Among Muslims, circumcision is called a *khitan* and is performed by an imam. There are regional differences in terms of the age at which the procedure is performed. It can be anywhere from shortly after birth to a bit before puberty.

Circumcision Through the Lens of an Anthropologist

This topic is very complex and could easily stand alone as a separate book. Broadly speaking, circumcision can mean different things to different people. In the United States, it is often seen as a normal part of infancy. In some cultures, it is seen as an initiation rite. It ensures social cohesion and helps an individual fully join their community (which is not necessarily a religious community). This can be observed in many parts of the world, from the United States to Africa to the South Pacific.

Circumcision Through the Lens of a Statistician

Most men in North America are circumcised men. In the United States, 79 percent of men do not have a foreskin. This percentage has, however, decreased over the last few decades. In fact, in the 1960s, 80 percent of newborns underwent the procedure; recent studies show only half of the male babies born in the United States are now being circumcised. In Canada, the percentage is much lower, at 48 percent.

In Europe, the countries of the former Yugoslavia have the highest percentages of circumcised men. In Albania, Bosnia and Herzegovina, and Macedonia, there are regions where up to 80 percent of the men are circumcised. The percentage of circumcised men in the rest of Europe is much lower, sitting around 20%. France is near the average, at 14 percent, while United Kingdom is quite a bit lower, at 9 percent. Denmark has the lowest rate of circumcised men, at 1.6 percent.

In Australia, 58 percent of men are circumcised. The percentage is much lower in New Zealand, where only 7 percent of newborn males undergo the procedure. This wasn't always the case, however. In the mid-20th century, 95 percent of newborn males were circumcised.

In Asia, circumcision depends largely on religious practice. While it is common in Muslim regions, it is rare, or very rare, outside of those communities. In Japan, only 1 perccent of men are circumcised.

Circumcision is very common in West Africa, with 90 percent of men having undergone the procedure. Elsewhere on the continent, Rwanda and South Africa have much lower percentages, with only 10 to 20 percent of men being circumcised.

Circumcision Through the Lens of a Mathematician

According to the World Health Organisation, 661 million men around the world are circumcised.

It is estimated that the weight (to be a true scientist, I should use the word mass) of a foreskin is around 0.07 ounces (2 g), which means that all of the foreskins that have been removed weigh a total of 4.66 billion ounces, 2,914,511 pounds or 1,457 tons (1.32 billion g, 1,322,000 kg or 1,322 metric tons).

An average semitrailer can carry about 30 tons, so almost 49 fully loaded semitrailers would be required to transport all of these removed foreskins. The average length of a semitrailer is about 50 feet (15 m), and it is not uncommon for traffic rules to dictate that drivers keep at least 160 feet (50 m) between two trucks. If the mathematician (me) is correct with his calculations, that convoy would be almost 2 miles (just over 3 km) long.

If you were to look out your window and watch these semitrailers go by at a city-driving speed of 30 miles per hour (50 km/h), you would be watching these foreskin-carrying trucks for about 4 minutes.

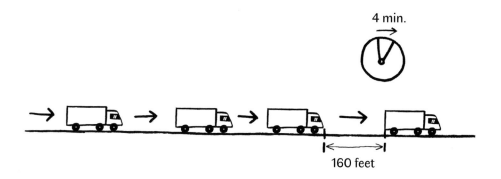

4 min.

160 feet

Circumcision Through the Lens of a Cosmetics Manufacturer

It is difficult to know the exact number of foreskins from circumcision operations that American hospitals sell to laboratories every year. Several years ago, a single foreskin could easily fetch between $35 and $50. These juvenile foreskins are valuable reservoirs of stem cells and fibroblasts, and labs use them as an ingredient in cosmetics. These creams and lotions are sold as antiaging, antiwrinkle or rejuvenating products. This is a lucrative business: A 1-ounce (28.4 g) bottle of TNS Essential Serum from SkinMedica costs $281.

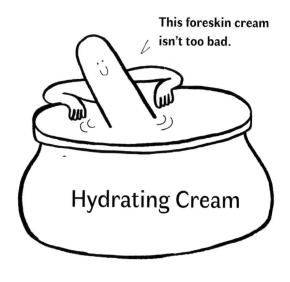

This foreskin cream isn't too bad.

Hydrating Cream

What Happens to a Foreskin Once It's Removed?

Jesus Christ was Jewish, so one can assume he was circumcised on the eighth day of his life. According to tradition, the removed foreskin was then buried. In the Middle Ages, however, several Christian sites claimed to possess the holy relic. In fact, at the time, there were no less than 14 sacred foreskins in Europe. However, that was a very special case. You may wonder what usually happens to foreskins, and that's a good question.

Among the Dii people, who live in the Adamawa region of northern Cameroon, young boys are circumcised. It is done with a yoob (spirit of the ancestors), which is a ritual knife. The removed foreskin is combined with a lion's heart and is used to make a stimulating mixture that is drunk by guests.

Circumcision is all but mandatory in Madagascar. An uncut man is often treated as an outcast by his community, and he will have great difficulty finding a companion. Once deceased, he is even buried away from others. Here, the removed foreskin is swallowed by the boy's grandfather: Nothing is created, nothing is lost, everything is transformed.

As previously noted, foreskins do not go to waste in the United States. They are collected and transformed by the cosmetics industry, and then people spread them on their face.

Can the Foreskin be Reconstructed?

Skin Grafts

There have been many attempts to reconstruct a foreskin with autologous skin grafts (taken from the patient himself). The skin must have a similar color and look, and it, of course, must be taken from an area that is completely hairless. This technique was abandoned due to disappointing results.

Non-surgical Techniques

There are several non-surgical procedures for reconstructing a foreskin, and all are based on gently and gradually elongating the skin.

Let's imagine a man who gains a lot of weight. His skin will expand as he does.

If this individual then loses weight and returns to his initial weight, his skin will not contract completely. It will stay about the same size and hang around him. This phenomenon is clearly visible in people who are morbidly obese and then lose a lot of weight. They often need to have surgery to remove the excess skin.

All of the non-surgical techniques use this characteristic of the skin. In practice, the area of skin located behind the glans penis is stretched. Traction should be gentle and painless but enough to be effective.

There are two challenges to overcome:

1. Gripping the skin: The simplest option is to hold the skin with medical glue or surgical tape, such as Micropore or Urgopore. There are also specially designed devices to help restore the foreskin. These use more sophisticated means to grip the skin, usually two small overlapping cups.

2. Gentle traction: It can be done very simply using tape, which is stretched before being applied to the skin. Commercial devices are also available, which use either a screw and nut system (such as the TLC-X device) or rubber bands (such as the DTR device). The TLC Tugger provides traction with an elastic strap, worn much like a sling.

These foreskin restoration systems are effective; they can rebuild an area of skin long enough to cover the glans and thus restore (to some extent) the foreskin. But don't be in hurry — it takes one to two years.

I say "to some extent" because these devices restore how the foreskin looks but not entirely how the original would have functioned. The neo-foreskin will lack the various sensory receptors that were present on the original, including Krause's corpuscles, which play a major role in how the brain perceives this area.

The Future: Grafting a Synthetic Foreskin

Research is being conducted by the Italian company Foregen with the goal of "repairing" circumcised men through regenerative medical procedures. It appears, however, that the research has come to a dead end.

A synthetic foreskin could be created with the following procedure: One must first obtain a matrix of the shape of the foreskin, without any foreign cells. This could be a foreskin from a cadaver that has been treated to eliminate the cells of the former owner or a laboratory-produced matrix made from collagen (which is the protein from which most organs are formed). Once this matrix is implanted, the recipient's cells would colonize it bit by bit. Once the foreskin is completely regenerated, it could be grafted onto the patient and would be completely accepted by his body since it would be composed of his own cells. No immunosuppressive therapy would be required.

A Penis Transplant?

"A woman's pleasure is not dependent upon the presence
of a penis in the vagina; neither is a man's."
— Germaine Greer

Autotransplantation is a transplant in which the donor and recipient
are the same person. It can involve, for example, a section of skin taken
from one area of the body and grafted onto another area. In terms of
the penis, it consists of reimplanting a penis that has been cut off. This
type of implantation poses no immune rejection problems since the
graft has the same immune characteristics as the rest of the body; there
is no risk of a person rejecting their own body part.

In allotransplantation, the graft comes from a donor who is the
same species as the recipient. In humans, the graft is taken from one
human and is transplanted to another human. In terms of immunity,
this transplant is different from the receiving body and will therefore

quickly be rejected, so the recipient must take antirejection medications for the rest of their life. This treatment decreases the recipient's immune defenses, so it is said to be immunosuppressive. While treatment is essential, it does carry risks. It can promote serious infections or even lead to the development of malignant tumors.

In xenotransplantation, the recipient and donor are different species. For example, transplanting a pig's kidney to a monkey or transplanting a chimpanzee's kidney to a human. (This type of transplantation really has been attempted.) Xenotransplantation poses significant rejection issues even with immunosuppressive therapy, and it is still in the experimental stages, with very few exceptions.

Penile Autotransplantation

Thailand holds an unenviable world record: It is the country with the most men who have had their penis cut off. Over the last three decades, more than 50 men have had their penis cut off, as compared to three in Sweden and two in the United States. The perpetrators have mostly been women, and they have not lacked imagination: the severed members were boiled, thrown in the garbage, thrown down a toilet, buried and even fed to ducks. One particularly inventive woman attached her husband's penis to a balloon and then let it fly away.

There is also a particularly distressing case that took place in China in 2015. A certain Mr. Fan had cheated on his wife with a certain Ms. Zhang, and his wife cut off his penis in anger. Fan's member was reimplanted, but his wife cut it off again, and this time it could not be recovered. Ms. Zhang was not too bothered, stating, "It doesn't matter that he's lost his fertility, he has five children already."

In most cases, however, a severed penis can be reimplanted.

Dr. Surasak Muangsombot, a Thai urologist at Paolo Memorial Hospital in Bangkok, is a penile reimplantation specialist. He advises that if a penis is amputated, it should immediately be put in a saline solution (available at pharmacies) at 39°F (4°C) in an insulated thermos and transporting it and the patient to a hospital.

Reimplantation consists of anastomosing (a medical term that simply means to connect) the different structures that we reviewed in the chapter on anatomy (see pages 12–21): the corpora cavernosa, corpus spongiosum, urethra, blood vessels, nerves and the skin. This is a very delicate surgery and is performed using a microscope. Results are generally good in terms of the survival of the transplanted member and the reestablishment of urinary evacuation but more mixed when it comes to sex, as only one in two patients regain the ability to have erections.

In the United States, John Wayne Bobbitt became infamous after having his penis cut off and then reattached. The resident of Manassas, Virginia, is alleged to have been violent toward his wife, and she, in a distressed state, cut off his penis. After his penis was successfully reimplanted, Bobbitt profited from his regained sexual ability by becoming a porn star. He was in the films *Uncut* and *Frankenpenis*. Inspired by the story, zoologists gave the common name Bobbit worm (with a single T) to the giant sea worm *Eunice aphroditois*, since the female is known to sever her partner's penis and eat it after they mate.

Penile Allotransplantation

Organ transplants (such as the heart, kidney and liver) are now commonplace, and the antirejection therapy is standardized and effective. Other transplants, such as face transplants, are much more difficult, since the graft is composed of different tissues: skin, muscle, bone, cartilage, etc. These more complex transplants are called composite grafts. On a technical level, they require many delicate sutures. Immunosuppressive therapy must also be potent, since composite grafts trigger more aggressive rejections than more straightforward organ transplants.

In the case of a penis, which is a composite organ, there is another particularity that delayed the first transplantation attempts. When it comes to a heart or a liver, the necessity of the operation isn't discussed because these are vital organs. However, the penis is not an organ that is necessary for life. This transplant therefore poses an ethical question: Is the risk of lifelong antirejection therapy worth the benefit of having a penis? There's another issue: Most recipients easily accept a deep organ transplant, such as a lung or kidney, but when it comes to a transplant that is more visible, such as a hand, the transplant recipient is sometimes unable to accept living with a "piece" of a deceased person in view. This lack of acceptance can quickly become a problem. For example, the first man to receive a hand transplant, in 1998, requested two and a half years later to have it amputated because he couldn't cope with having a foreign hand.

A Chinese team performed the first penis transplant on September 21, 2005. The recipient was a 44-year-old man who had lost his member due to lower abdominal trauma from a car crash. The donor was a 22-year-old who was brain dead. The surgical team was led by Dr. Weilie Hue and performed the operation at a hospital in Guangzhou. The procedure lasted 15 hours, and there were no postoperative problems. However, 14 days later, the recipient requested to have his new member amputated because he could not handle having the penis of a deceased man.

It wasn't until December 11, 2014, that Dr. Frank Graewe and his team performed the second penis implant, at Tygerberg Hospital in Cape Town, South Africa. The recipient was a 21-year-old man who had lost his penis due to gangrene following a ritual circumcision. The donor was a 36-year-old man. The patient quickly regained his urinary and sexual functions, and he had sex only a week after he left the hospital. He even became a father the following year. The donor was a white man and the recipient was a person of color. Recent reports are suggesting he plans to have his transplanted organ tattooed to match the rest of his body.

The third penis transplant took place in the United States on May 8, 2016. Dr. Curtis Cetrulo led a team at Massachusetts General Hospital and transplanted a penis onto Thomas Manning, a man who had his own removed as part of penile cancer treatment.

Again in the United States, another surgical team, led by Dr. Andrew Lee at John Hopkins Hospital, achieved a world first: a transplantation of both a penis and a scrotum. The recipient was a soldier who had been injured by an improvised explosive device in Afghanistan. The scrotum did not include the testicles, to prevent the patient from procreating with the donor's sperm, which would pose obvious ethical problems.

The Future: Artificial Penis Transplants

Penis transplants are clearly not the stuff of legend. Every year, men lose their penis to cancer treatment, infections or accidents. There are also many victims whose genitals are mutilated from war injuries, and it is estimated that in the United States alone, 100 soldiers have been disfigured in this way during the Afghanistan and Iraq wars. Furthermore, these injuries are very hard to deal with psychologically, and many of the injured commit suicide.

As with other transplants, there is a shortage of donors. This shortage is even more acute than for other organs, since females cannot contribute, and it is preferable, for psychological reasons, that the donor and recipient have the same skin color. To address this situation, researchers are developing an artificial penis. The Wake Forest Institute for Regenerative Medicine (WFIRM), famous for creating the first implantable artificial human bladder in 1999, has been studying for over 20 years now the production of an artificial penis.

The process would be as follows: Researchers first create a collagen mold of the penis (collagen is a structural protein, meaning it forms the framework of organs). They then take cells from the recipient, multiply these in a culture and then place them in the mold. These cells would then colonize and grow the desired organ bit by bit. The big advantage is that this synthetic organ would be accepted by the recipient's immune system, since it would be made of his own cells. Therefore, antirejection therapy would not be required. One drawback, however, is that an artificial penis would be made up of several types of tissues, so its production is much more complex than an organ that is not composite, such as the bladder.

WFIRM's research is at an advanced stage, and they have been developing implantable penises for rabbits since 2008. These penises were transplanted onto 12 rabbits. Afterward, female rabbits were presented to the rabbits who had received a transplanted penis. Eight of the male rabbits were able to ejaculate and four had offspring.

What About Penile Xenotransplantation?

In the 1920s, a French surgeon of Russian origin, Serge Voronoff, tried to rejuvenate aging men by transplanting sections of chimpanzee testicles into these men's scrotums. He thereby accumulated a sizable fortune.

During this same era in the United States, John Romulus Brinkley was transplanting goat testicles into men who had a low sex drive. In 16 years, he performed transplants on more than 5,000 men. The only result was a placebo effect, since those testicle transplants did not survive. Each operation cost $750, which at the time was very expensive, and Brinkley became one of the richest men in the country.

Why stop at testicles? Now we wait for an inventive surgeon to transplant an animal penis onto a man...

Penis Apparel

There are many kinds of "clothing" for the penis. Some are purely decorative, while others keep it warm, and others still are just neat gadgets. And, of course, some offer erotic enjoyment. Let's look at what has been invented since man took an interest in his member and sought to dress it up.

Codpiece

In the 16th century, every trendy man wore a codpiece. It was a piece of triangular cloth that was worn over the crotch. It was originally a simple length of cloth fastened with straps or buttons that was meant to cover the genitals, but its role quickly evolved. Rather than hide the genitals, it was used to attract attention to the area.

To provide flattering volume to the wearer's, ahem, attributes, the codpiece was padded and became increasingly prominent. To make things even more eye catching, the padding was arranged in such a way that it gave the appearance that the gussied-up man had a permanent erection. Numerous portraits of the era show men in codpieces.

Even suits of armor were equipped with codpieces, made from bulging metal shells. Some examples have survived to this day: Emperor Ferdinand I's armor with codpiece can be seen at the Metropolitan Museum of Art in New York, and Henry VIII's equally flattering armor is displayed at the Tower of London.

Chastity Cage

This device, intended for the those who partake in BDSM (which stands for bondage, discipline, sadism and masochism), comes in metal and various colors of plastic. It is composed of two parts. A ring firmly encloses the base of the scrotum, which prevents the device from being taken off, and a perforated casing, which allows urine to pass through, slides over the penis. The two parts can be joined by a chain, which prevents the wearer from getting an erection.

Chastity garments, however, are not new. Cluny Museum in France has a chastity belt for women that not only protected the vulva but would surely have kept out even the best escape artists. This belt allowed defecation only through a small cutout in the shape of a clover. You can imagine how the resultant material must have looked after having traveled through that passage, not to mention the suffering of the unfortunate women locked up in such a way!

Protective Cup

Even when playing non-contact sports, athletes can occasionally be subjected to very violent blows to their genitals, either from a ball or a mishap. The consequences range from simple pain to serious lesions, which can include ruptured testicles or a crushed penis. Wearing a protective cup helps limit the risks. They are generally made from durable plastic, and their shape helps contain the penis and scrotum. The most comfortable kinds have flexible walls or a soft gel edge. Cups are generally designed to be worn with specially adapted underwear or an athletic supporter.

Penile Sheath

This penis "garment," also called a *koteka* or *horim*, is worn by certain Indigenous peoples in New Guinea. The penis is inserted into a long gourd and kept in place by tying vegetable fibers around the scrotum. Some *koteka* are decorated with carvings or even shells or feathers. Seeking to modernize their society or perhaps bowing to the pressures of Westernization, the local government tried, in vain, to stop men from wearing *koteka*. They have now settled on requiring men to wear shorts to enter official buildings.

Medical Penile Sheath

This device is intended for men who are suffering from urinary incontinence. It is made from a latex sheath and is about as thick as a condom, and it fits snugly on the penis. This sheath has an extended tip that can be connected to a tube that leads to a colostomy bag. There are colostomy bags that can be attached to the leg, which give wearers some autonomy throughout the day, and there are larger capacity bags for overnight use. Some manufacturers also offer penile sheaths for short penises (2 inches / 5 cm).

Silicone Extender

Silicone is a plastic material that has many advantages, including being well tolerated by the body. For that reason, the Asian company Sexy-Fun chose it as the material from which to make their "reusable extension sleeves for men." There are two types: small and large.

The small sleeve is shaped like an elongated glans and is around 2 inches (5 cm) long. It is hollow and slips onto the real glans, which gives the penis an extra inch or so of length. The manufacturer's product guide provides the following information:

This product is not a contraceptive. Gives women more intense stimulation. Can be reused.

The second model comes as a well-sized erect penis and is also hollow. It slips on like a glove. The description states:

Hollow reservoir tip ensures suction cup fit that grips right on to you.

Here we are reassured that we are not likely to lose it in the vagina during the heat of the moment. As for the results, the website promises that dots and embossments on the surface mimic blood vessels, providing better stimulation for a lady's G-spot.

Dots and similar to the blood vessels embossment on the surface for better stimulation your ladies G-spot.

High-Fashion Penis

Rick Owens is an American fashion designer who turned heads when he showed his autumn-winter 2015 menswear collection. The models walked out in clothing with cut-outs that left their penises exposed. Some spectators were offended, not because of the nudity, but because the unfortunate models were "shriveled." This was most likely the effects of stress; it can't be easy to strut your stuff in such clothing in front of a few hundred people. In the weeks following the runway, the designer was nicknamed Dick Owens.

Kynodesme

Nudity was more accepted in ancient Greece than it is today. Showing your penis was widely accepted, especially during sporting events, fights or even during certain theatrical performances. However, each era has its prohibitions, and while showing one's penis was not typically problematic, it was considered to be in very bad taste to show off the tip: the glans penis. Ancient Greeks were of the opinion that only slaves and barbarians displayed this appendage. The *kynodesme* was invented to keep the glans out of sight.

Etymologically, *kynodesme* literally means "dog leash," which is fitting, since it is a leather cord. One end was tied around the foreskin, and the other end was attached to a leather strap that circles the waist. This assembly lifted the penis, which not only hid the glans but exposed the scrotum, which was quite fashionable. What's more, the foreskin was pulled up, which tends to lengthen it; for the ancient Greeks, having a long foreskin was aesthetically pleasing. Subsequently, the Etruscans and then the Romans adopted the *kynodesme* and latinizing its name, and this accessory became known as the *ligature praeputii*.

Cologne

In a 1960 interview with Marie Claire magazine, Norma Jeane Mortenson said:

What do I wear to bed? Chanel N° 5.

That Norma Jeane Mortenson wears neither pajamas nor a nightgown to bed and just a few drops of a well-known fragrance matters very little to us. Although perhaps that changes if we specify she is better known by the name Marilyn Monroe.

Recently, men also have a fragrance that they can wear to "dress up" for bed. Better still, this cologne is specially formulated for the penis, hence it merits a mention in this book.

It is called FresHim. This product comes in a spray, and the maker recommends spraying it in the morning and evening at a distance of about 4 inches (10 cm) from the penis. They claim that not only will FresHim have your penis smelling great, it also acts as a deodorizer. Better still, the cherry — or glans, rather — on the sundae is that FresHim will keep your penis healthy because it contains provitamin B5, vitamin E and aloe vera.

Condoms

There's so much to write about condoms that the topic deserves its own book. Let's settle on pointing out a few little-known facts. For example, the materials that condoms are made from. The very first ones, which can be traced back to the time of the Egyptian pyramids, were simply a sheep caecum (which is sheep intestine; this material was used because it naturally had a handy dead end). Later, condoms were made of velvet, oiled canvas or silk for the most luxurious experience. They were specifically designed to prevent conception as well as to protect the wearer from venereal diseases. Today, most condoms are made from latex, and synthetic rubber condoms are available for people with latex allergies. There are even condoms designed for fellatio lovers that are available in strawberry, banana or mint flavors, and it seems that there will soon be shrimp-flavored ones. Lastly, for those who are afraid of the dark, there are glow-in-the-dark condoms.

TUX

The Swedish site lelo.com, an online store specializing in all types of erotic gadgets, claims to sell the very first tuxedo for penises. It comes in one size, but Lelo advises it can stretch to fit all shapes and sizes. It is all satin, including the bow tie. Final point: it should be taken off in the event of sexual intercourse. It seems that TUX was designed to help your penis look fancy but not to prevent pregnancy or the spread of disease. Younger readers will be happy to know that Lelo offers a 15 percent student discount.

Willy Warmer

A kilt is a traditional Scottish garment. Scotland, however, has a rather cold climate, and tradition excludes the wearing of underwear, which is considered too modern. So how do the kilt-donning Scots keep their penis from getting cold? The answer is simple: a wool willy warmer. This knitted cover can be slipped over the penis to protect it from the cold.

Designed for comfort, it even has a slightly wider pocket for warming the wearer's testicles. Similar items can be found in other cold and mountainous regions, including Croatia's Mrkopalj region, the Faroe Islands (where it is known as a *kallvøttur*) and Norway (where it's called a *voenakot*). In the case of Norway, the warmest types are made with squirrel fur — on the inside, of course.

If you live in a cold climate and don't know how to knit and squirrels are scarce, you can buy a willy warmer online. You can find different types starting at around $10. They're available in a range of colors and are guaranteed not to shrink.

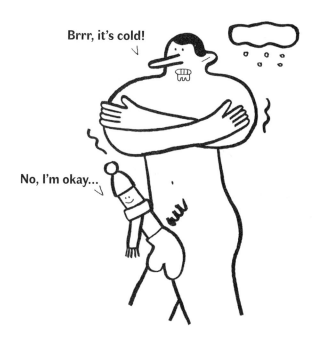

Can You Eat A Penis?

"I ate his liver with some fava beans and a nice chianti."
— **Thomas Harris**, *The Silence of the Lambs*

You Can Eat It with Brussels Sprouts

Vorarephilia is a rare sexual deviation, or paraphilia, to use the proper psychiatric term, that involves experiencing sexual arousal from the idea of either eating one's partner or being eaten by them. Like many sexual deviations, it does not really pose any problems as long as it remains a fantasy. But it becomes problematic when the fetishizer starts firing up the stove and writes a post to find fresh meat.

The ad "Looking for a young man, 18–30 years old, well-built, for slaughter," posted in 2001 on an online dating site, helped Armin Meiwes, a German computer technician, find a partner named Bernd Jürgen Brandes to have sex with, initially. That's not a big deal. However, Meiwes's true objective was to satisfy his cannibalistic desires, which is significantly more worrisome. Branders's penis was cut off, fried and eaten by both lovers. Meiwes killed Bernd, carved a steak from out of his back and ate it with a side of brussels sprouts. At his trial, he said the first bite was very strange, and explained how he had been waiting for that moment for 40 years. He said it tasted like pork, but richer.

You Can Eat It
with Mushrooms and Parsley

More recently, in 2012, Japanese artist Mao Sugiyama who considers themself asexual, was surgically castrated and invited five people to a restaurant in Suginami to eat their genitals, which would be cooked with mushrooms and parsley. The artist had taken the precaution of producing a medical certificate stating that they were free of any vene-real disease and had guests sign a contract attesting that they were

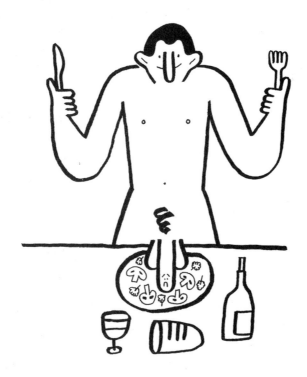

going to consume human flesh with full knowledge of the facts. Sugiyama was subsequently prosecuted, but the charges were dropped because, strangely enough, cannibalism is not illegal in Japan.

Recipes

Tunisian Jews have developed a dish called *akod* that is made from the tripe and penis of an ox. It is seasoned with cumin and paprika. You can find recipes online.

The Chinese also have a few dishes that contain the penis of an animal. On such dish is crocodile penis soup.

Special Vegan Version

Vegans do not use or consume any animal products. Penis, therefore, is definitely not on their menu. Luckily for foodies, there's a vegan alternative: a mushroom.

My father was an amateur mycologist, and his hobby was to walk through the woods foraging for rare or little-known mushrooms, identify them and, if possible, eat them. From time to time, he would bring me along, and one day I spotted a strange growth sticking out of the ground. It was a *Phallus impudicus*. As its name suggests, this mushroom resembles an erect penis. What's more, it emits a very strong odor intended to attract flies, which help disperse its spores.

Coming back to our topic, this phallic mushroom is edible, at least while it's still in its early stages of growth and the smell is still bearable. According to Lithuanian researchers, it even has anticancer properties. If you'd like to try to grow your own *Phallus impudicus*, there are retailers who sell its mycelium online (it's also known as the common stinkhorn).

How the Sausage Gets Made

Several years ago, I asked a patient who was a butcher what happens to the pigs' genitals at his shop. Do they get thrown out? Are they used for something? He told me they were not thrown out but were used to make pâté and were simply mixed in with "everything else." Goes to show that everything has its use.

Penis Hygiene

Smegma

In medical terms, this substance is said to be caseous, which is from the Latin *caseum*, meaning cheese. The term describes its appearance. Almost all mammals, including humans, produce smegma.

The preputial glands, as their name suggests, are found on the inside of the prepuce, or foreskin. In uncircumcised men these glands are largely hidden. They should not be confused with the small, visible bumps that sometimes appear around the base of the glans, known as pearly penile papules, which are sebaceous glands (they secrete sebum, which is an oily film that protects the skin). Smegma is produced when the secretions of the preputial glands mixes with dead skill cells from the surface of the foreskin. This yellowish-white substance can accumulate between the glans penis and the foreskin, especially at the balano-preputial fold.

Circumcised men produce very little to no smegma, which makes sense, since they no longer have a foreskin. The production of smegma varies depending on age. There is very little in infants, a little more in children, and production increases significantly as puberty begins. Production is highest around 24 years old and then decreases, often disappearing completely in middle-aged men. Females also produce smegma. It can be found under the clitoral hood and where the labia minora and labia majora meet.

Contrary to a long-held belief, the presence of smegma is not a sign of disease; it is completely physiological and can even be useful — nature does nothing in vain. It serves several purposes

- In early childhood, smegma lubricates the area where the glans penis meets the foreskin, facilitating the unhooding of the foreskin when it's time to go to the bathroom or when handling the penis. This unhooding, which will naturally happen from time to time (never do it with force!), can help prevent the onset of phimosis.
- Later in life, smegma plays a lubricating role during sex.
- In many animals, smegma contains volatile substances that produce an odor: pheromones. They play a role in sexual behavior. It is very likely that the same is true in humans, albeit to a lesser degree.

This discussion of pheromones reminds me of a tale a Don Juan type once told me. When he was looking to attract someone, he would take a bit of his own smegma and rub it behind his ears and on his neck. This seductor told me that this process makes the man irresistible in the eyes (or rather the nose?) of any woman, making it much easier to seduce her. I am willing to believe him, considering his many conquests.

Some doctors have wondered whether the presence of smegma is associated with penile cancers or even cervical cancers in women. Human papillomavirus infection is most likely the main cause of penile cancer, but the American Cancer Society does list phimosis and smegma as risk factors.

When smegma is left for too long, bacteria often develop, and the smegma produces a strong, unpleasant odor. You may be tempted to wash until you eliminate the odor entirely, since by today's standards "clean" means odorless. In the past, smells of everyday life, including body odors, were pervasive across all segments of society and likely reached such an intensity that it would certainly be difficult to bear them with our modern noses. If we could travel back in time, training for time travelers would almost certainly include, among other things, getting accustomed to invasive smells.

However, we live in the present. Unless you live alone in the middle of the woods, it's not possible to let odors develop from your genitals by never washing them and leaving them coated in a thick layer of smegma, which will certainly become very stinky over time. Smegma is, however, a useful substance. It's not a matter of aggressively cleansing with soap or shower gel two, three or more times a day to try to eliminate the slightest trace. It suffices to wash the area regularly.

Let's now return to the initial topic, about bacteria and microbes. Since first being discovered by Louis Pasteur, bacteria and microbes are well known if not, perhaps, always fully understood. Until recently, bacteria were universally and indiscriminately considered bad and dangerous, since they were regarded as causing illnesses.

To maintain their good health, people often assumed they had to eliminate as many bacteria and microbes as possible, hence the success of advertisements for cleaning products boasting that they can eliminate 99.9% of bacteria. However, recent and quite robust studies have redefined our perceptions of microbiota. This shift is a major advance in understanding our interactions with bacteria and other viruses.

Microbiota

The first studies that demonstrated the beneficial effects of microbes in the human body studied intestinal flora. These studies demonstrated that the immune system cannot mature properly if the subject's intestines are completely devoid of bacteria. Intestinal bacteria provide many benefits, since they compete against other significantly more pathogenic bacteria, protecting the body from infections. A "good" microbiota can also help prevent diabetes, allergies and obesity. All these beneficial microbes make up what is called gut microbiota.

Researchers quickly realized that there were other microbes located on the skin, in the nose and mouth, and around the genitals. The glans penis and foreskin area have their own microbiota, which provides protection similar to that provided by a healthy gut microbiata. This microflora must therefore be respected.

To air out this chapter, if you will, here is an interesting story from my many years of practice as a general practitioner. A female patient of mine was brought up in a strict household and demanded impeccable cleanliness, especially with regards to her genitals. This 40-year-old woman would pop into the bathroom four to five times a day to scrub her vulva with soap.

This patient complained of severe irritation of her genitals. I examined her more than once, but the examinations didn't reveal anything, although she sometimes had mycosis. With much difficulty, I managed to convince her to stop her excessive washing, and soon after she no longer had any issues. In short, hygiene is necessary, but not excessively so!

The Aging Penis

**"We don't stop playing because we grow old.
We grow old because we stop playing."
— George Bernard Shaw**

With age, the skin sags, hair falls out and turns white, muscles lose their strength, and memory weakens. But what becomes of the penis?

The Skin

Penis skin, like the skin on the rest of the body, thins and becomes more fragile with age. When injured, skin can also take longer to heal. Hair falls out over time and can even almost disappear with old age, and what remains turns gray or white.

A person with an aging penis may be tempted to use dye to rejuvenate his hair down there. This cover-up may seem like a good idea to prepare for an encounter with a new partner, but it is best to avoid using hair dye because there is a significant risk of irritation and the color fades. Henna is also strongly discouraged because it can lead to severe local reactions. There are specially formulated products for dyeing hair in sensitive areas that do not contain ammonia and are not likely to irritate the skin. These dyes come in black, brown and blond.

Looking for something more interesting? Why not dare to go blue, purple, orange or neon pink? These dyes are also available.

Size

For most men, the penis tends to shrink with age. It is estimated that this loss is on average 0.5 inches (1 cm) per decade from the age of 40. This decrease can be due to the scarcity or absence of sex for some men. In addition, a buried penis may cause such "shrinkage." This is an accumulation of fat in the abdominal and pelvic regions, common in men of a certain age, which leads to a visible, but not actual, decrease in penis length. This phenomenon is discussed in the chapter dedicated to penis size (see pages 38–60).

Function and Performance

It's no secret that a man's sexual performance often diminishes as he ages. Erections are not as frequent, and while previously the mere mention of an erotic situation could ensure rigidity, as he ages a real-life scenario will be required to achieve the same result, and later still oral or manual stimulation may become necessary.

This decrease in performances is due to an array of interconnected factors:

- Lower testosterone levels: This hormone is secreted in large quantities during puberty, reaches its peak between the ages of 20 and 30 years and then levels begin to decrease in one's 60s to about half of what they were in one's 30s. It can be tempting to administer this hormone to restore blood levels — we will explore this a little later on in this section.

- Atherosclerosis: With age, arteries begin to degrade due to high blood pressure, high levels of certain lipids and especially diabetes. Atherosclerosis can cause a stroke or heart attack, but it can also affect a person's sex life. Inadequate blood supply affects the quality of erections, and advanced atherosclerosis can cause ED. It is commonly held that the ability to maintain good quality erections with age confirms good cardiovascular health.
- Fibrosis of the tunica albuginea: This envelope that contains the corpora cavernosa can be gradually taken over by fibrous tissue. It becomes less stretchy and can begin to obstruct erections.
- Cerebral aging and low sex drive: Conventional wisdom, in both a medical and popular sense, often affirms, with reason, that our sexual organ is found between our ears.

The refractory period will also increase. The refractory period is the time it takes a man to achieve a new erection after sex with ejaculation. In very young men, the refractory period is short and generally lasts less than 10 minutes. In older men, it can be several hours or even a day. Refractory periods are further discussed in the chapter dedicated to erections (see page 31).

Is This Andropause?

Until recently, it was common to group the different disorders in men of a certain age under the term "andropause," which served as an analog to menopause, which happens to middle-aged women. Andropause, however, is not the correct term.

Menopause is characterized by a major drop in hormonal secretions in the female body. Symptoms can appear quickly and are sometimes intense. In men, hormonal secretions decrease very gradually, and health problems develop in a much more insidious way. Hence the recent concept of androgen deficiency in the aging male (ADAM).

Androgen Deficiency in the Aging Male (ADAM)

ADAM requires two conditions:
1. The patient must have a combination of certain well-identified disorders and these must significantly impair his quality of life
2. Testosterone levels in blood serum must be low

First, we'll look at the relevant disorders and then what to make of the testosterone serum levels.

ADAM Symptoms

Men with androgen deficiency generally complain about the following problems:
- Low sex drive
- Decrease in spontaneous nocturnal and morning erections
- Unsatisfactory erections or even absence of erections despite partner stimulation
- Significant increase in the length of the refractory period
- Hot flashes
- Night sweats
- Difficulty sleeping, with frequent nighttime awakenings

- Memory lapses
- Lack of attention
- Fatigue
- Sleepiness after meals
- Lack of vitality
- Depressed mood

It is worth noting that apart from the so-called climacteric disorders (hot flashes, sweats), these disorders are either sexual or psychological in nature. However, everyone has suffered from memory lapses, lack of attention, a low moment or a sexual breakdown at some point in their life. For an ADAM diagnosis, a man must present clear episodes of several of these disorders, and the disorders should be permanent. It is estimated that a quarter of men have ADAM after age 50, and half have it at age 70. Obesity and chronic alcoholism are risk factors for ADAM.

Signs That Can Be Observed by a Doctor

- Abdominal obesity; while it may sound a bit crass, it paints a picture: it's said that the patient can't see himself pee anymore
- Hair loss on the the armpits, pubis, legs and, to a lesser extent, the face
- Thin and fragile skin
- Decrease in muscle mass in all four limbs
- Decrease in testicular volume

A Self-Assessment to Screen for ADAM

The *Metabolism 2000* journal published a 10-point questionnaire to help men self-screen for ADAM. Here it is:

1. Do you have a decrease in libido (sex drive)?
2. Do you have a lack of energy?
3. Do you have a decrease in strength and/or endurance?
4. Have you lost height?
5. Have you noticed a decrease in your enjoyment of life?
6. Are you sad and/or grumpy?
7. Are your erections less strong?
8. Have you noticed a recent deterioration in your ability to play sports?
9. Are you falling asleep after dinner?
10. Has your work performance recently declined?

According to the questionnaire's authors, if you answered yes to question 1 or 7 or if you answer yes to at least three questions, it is likely that you have ADAM. In that case, you should discuss taking a testosterone level test with your doctor.

However, an assessment such as this one is open to criticism because if we take a step back, we realize that the authors' questions are quite broad.

Blood Testosterone Level

Put somewhat simply, testosterone exists in the blood in two forms. One type is tied to a protein and is not directly usable by the organs. The other type is called free testosterone because it is directly usable by organs. With age, there is a small change in the total level of testosterone in the blood, but the level of free testosterone decreases significantly. Thus, it is the free testosterone that needs to be measured. The level of testosterone in the blood varies throughout the day, so it should be measured in the morning between 8 a.m. and 10 a.m.

Normal values depend on the laboratory and are provided with the results. Here are typical values:

- Between 36 and 50 years old: 0.8–3.2 ng/ml
- Between 51 and 70 years old: 0.3–2.9 ng/ml

Diagnosis

When considering an ADAM diagnosis, the challenge is distinguishing between what is physiological (everyone ages and everyone loses their abilities) and what is genuinely abnormal or pathological. The doctor must consider how the patient feels. You don't simply treat blood levels for a hormone that is too low, you care for a person and try to provide them relief. Thus, it is essential to assess the patient's discomfort. Many of the disorders attributed to ADAM can also be attributed to hypothyroidism; it's necessary to eliminate that diagnosis.

Assessment Before Treatment

Prostate cancer is a common cancer in older men. Data from routine autopsies show that there are small cancer sites in one-third of men aged 50 to 59 years old. Half of men in their 60s are carriers, and all men in their 80s are carriers. I say "carriers" here and not men "with cancer" because the presence of these sites does not mean that all of these men were sick. In most cases, these prostate cancer sites do not evolve, or they evolve so slowly that their carrier dies from something else completely. It's important to know about the common presence of prostate cancer because it is a hormone-dependent cancer, which means that the growth is stimulated by testosterone. The higher the level of the hormone, the higher the risk of developing an active cancer, causing disorders.

Because treatment for ADAM is based on administering testosterone, it is necessary to ensure the patient does not have a detectable prostate cancer before starting it. In practice, the doctor requests a blood test to obtain the level of a prostate-specific antigen (PSA; levels become elevated with prostate cancer) and will conduct a digital rectal exam to look for a nodule or suspected area. These two associated tests help detect many but not all tumors.

Another cancer that needs to be screened for is breast cancer. It does not occur exclusively in females; 1 percent of mammary tumors affect men. This cancer is also hormone-dependent, but in this case, estrogens promote growth. A history of such cancer prohibits any testosterone treatment. This can seem illogical, since testosterone is a male hormone, but in the body, aromatase (an enzyme) transforms testosterone into estrogen. A breast exam is done before the initiation of the treatment for ADAM.

The last indisputable contraindication to starting a testosterone treatment is a history of sexual offenses. It is logical to prohibit testosterone treatment in this case because it will increase sex drive and the ability to get an erection; consequently, it increases the risk of a new offense.

Testosterone is also known to increase the production of red blood cells. It is therefore not advisable to administer it if the patient already has too many red blood cells (polycythemia), since it increases the risk of thrombosis. Similarly, the existence of other risk factors of thrombosis should encourage caution but does not formally prohibit treatment.

Benign prostatic hyperplasia (BHP) is common at the age when most men are diagnosed with ADAM. Testosterone can aggravate urinary disorders due to BHP, so it is necessary to weigh the pros and cons for each patient before initiating treatment.

Treatment

Simply put, treatment consists of administering testosterone, which can be done three ways:

- Intramuscular delivery via injections
- Oral delivery via tablets or capsules
- Transdermal delivery via gels or patches

These drugs are applied by the patients themselves. In the case of a gel, under no circumstances should a female partner handle them, to ensure she does not inadvertently absorb some of the hormone. The gel is spread over the arms and shoulders (never on the genitals), and it is necessary to wait several minutes for the gel to penetrate the skin before getting dressed. These treatments are relatively new, and we are still learning much about ADAM and how best to treat it. Consult your doctor if you have concerns about your testosterone levels and what treatments, if any, are appropriate.

Treatment Monitoring

Monitoring is essential. It is recommended to assess patients in the third, sixth and twelfth month and yearly thereafter. There are three components:

- An interview to assess mood and look for possible adverse effects (especially irritability and urinary discomfort)
- A clinical exam, including blood pressure measurement, breast exam and rectal exam
- Blood work, including a testosterone level, blood count (to look for polycythemia) and PSA test. If an increase in PSA is found, it is imperative to conduct further examination to look for possible prostate cancer.

Results

I've renewed and monitored the treatments for several men with ADAM using testosterone via transdermal delivery, and I've noticed that this treatment significantly improves their quality of life. Sex becomes more satisfying and, like women taking hormone replacement therapy, these patients remain dynamic and have a good morale. This treatment is therefore important, but it is far from being harmless.

What To Call It

General

Baby Bazooka
Bagpipe
Banger
Bedfellow
Beef Bayonet
Beef Bullet
Big One
Bollocks
Captain Kielbasa
Cock-hammer
Cockerel
Cocktapus
Crack Pipe
Dick Hardington
Dipstick
Dodger
Dong
Doodle
Dr. Orgazmo
Erector Set

Family Jewels
Family Organ
Fixed Bayonet
Flapdoodle
Gadget
Gear
Giblets
Happy Handle
Hard-on
Jack
Jackhammer
Jock and Roll
Jock Monster
Joystick
King Dong
Kit
Knacker
Knick-Knacks
Lance
Lance Corporal
Lap Rocket

Leather Hose
Leather Stretcher
Longfellow
Louisville Slugger
Love Auger
Love Hammer
Love Musket
Magnum P.I.
Man Meat
Man Muscle
Man Root
Manhood
Marriage Tackle
Meat Mallet
Meat Whistle
Mr. Happy
Ol'Baldy
One-eyed Wonder
Organ Grinder
Patootie
Pee-wee

Peenchuck
Peeshooter
Poker
Pump Handle
Rock Hammer
Shaft
Staff Member
Steak and Eggs
Tallywag
Tan Banana
Third Arm
Third Leg
Tootsie Pop
Vlad the Impaler
Weenie
Whackhammer
Whanger
Womb Broom
Womb Raider
Zipper Dipper
Zipper Kipper
Zipper Ripper
Zipper Skipper
Zipper Whipper

Traditional
Choad
Chub
Chubby
Cock
Cockstand
Ding-a-ling
Dingle
Dingus

Dingy
Dink
Dork
Pecker
Peen
Pizzle
Prick
Pud
Pudge
Wick

One of the boys
Able Seaman
Action Jackson
Dick
Jimbo
John Thomas
Johnson
Old Boy
One-eyed Pete
Peter
Rod
Roger
Willy

Yiddish
Putz
Schlong
Schmeckel (a boy's)
Schmuck
Schwantz
Shtupper

Lunch
Bone
Dicksicle
Hog
Hot Dog
Kielbasa
Meat and 2 vegetables
Meat Puppet
Noodle
Osca Wee-wee
Pickle
Porker
Purple Pickle
Root
Salami
Snausage
Tube Steak

Hardware
Ball Peen
Crank
Drill
Extendo
Hammer
Hose
Junk
Knob
Maypole
Member
Package
Plunger
Pocket Rocket
Rod and Reel

Tackle
Thwacker
Tool
Unit
Wand
Wood
Woody
Wrench

Wild Kingdom

Baloney Pony
Chunky Monkey
Donkey Dong
Drillosaurus
Hairy Canary
One-eyed Snake
Pant Python
Purple Python
Trouser Monkey
Trouser Snake

Romantic

Baby-maker
Love Gun
Love Muscle
Purple Love Stick
Sex Pistol
Whoopie Stick
Womb Broom

Descriptors

Disco Stick
Kilt Wicket
One-eyed Monster

Pipe Organ
Purple Cigar
Skin Flute

Misc

Pee-Pee
Peggo
Pillicock
Pintle
Plonker
Runnion
Tallywhacker
Wee-Wee
Wingwang
Winkie

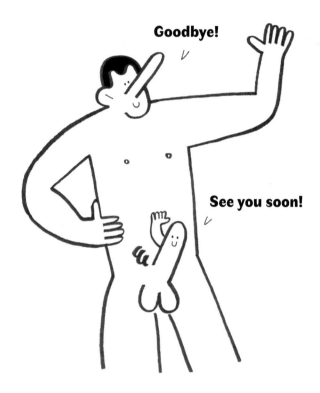

Index

meatotomy 146
meatus, urinary *see* urinary meatus
Medicated Urethral System for Erection (MUSE) 131–132
megaphallus 98–99
melanin 19–21 84–85
melanocytes 19–21, 84
microbiota 77, 188–189
microphallus 49, 53, 57–59, 62, 73–74
mites 89–90
mohel 160
MRI of penis 21
MUSE *see* Medicated Urethral System for Erection

N
Naga Baba sect (India) 66
Napoleon 57–58
necrosis 65, 149
Neotragla species 27–28
nerves
erector 128
pelvic splanchnic 32
nitric oxide (NO) 32, 34–35, 134–135, 138
nocturnal erections 36, 193
non-ischemic priapism 104, 105, 153–154

O
obesity
ADAM and 194
erectile dysfunction and 117
octopus 23, 28
odaxelagnia 99
odor 79–80
cologne, penile 179
pheromones 15
smegma 77, 102, 186–188
oetang *150, 151*
oral sex 83, 90, 110–111, 180
orgasm 36
Owens, Rick 178

P
papaverine 104, 129
paper nautilus 23
paraphimosis 100, 102, 157l
see also phimosis
parasites 86, 89–90

passive erection 126, 128
pearls, penile 148–149
pearly penile papules 17–18, 186
pelvic splanchnic nerve 32
penectomy 146–148
penicillin 81–82
penile adhesions 16, 77
retractile 107–108
penile dysmorphic disorder 63
penile strangulation 154–155
penis captivus 101
penoplasty 70–74, 71
Peyronie's disease 95–97
Phallus impudicus 184–185
pheromones 15, 187
phimosis 16, 102–103, 157, 158, 187; *see also* paraphimosis
phosphodiesterase type 5 (PDE5) 33, 35, 124–125
phytoestrogens 92
piercings 149–151, *150*
Ponchietti R., 43
pornography 39, 44, 56, 57, 63, 86, 169
posthectomy *see* circumcision
posthitis 102
preputial glands 159, 186
preputial ring 16, 102, 158, 159; *see also* foreskin
preputioplasty 103, 158–159
priapism 54–55, 104–105, 130, 137, 154, 155
Prince Albert (piercing) *150, 151*
protective cup 176
puberty 12–13, 16, 18, 20, 53, 62
pubic bone 14, *15, 71*
pumps 68, 78, 126–128, *127, 128, 133,* 133–134

R
Rasputin 53, 53–54
reduction, penile 98–99
refractory period 36, 192, 193
reimplantation, penis 167–169; *see also* transplant, penile
religious requirements for circumcision 160

retrograde ejaculation 126, 154
reverse Prince Albert (piercing) *150,* 151

S
Sarcoptes scabiei hominis 89–90
scabies 89–90
scrotum 140, 171, 173, 179
sebaceous glands 12, 16, 186
semen *see* sperm
severed penis 168–169
sex drive 173, 192, 193
sexual anxiety 119
sexually transmitted diseases (STD) 81–83, 89–90
sexually transmitted infections (STI) 81, 83–84, 90–91, 108–111, 156–157
sheath, penile 176–177
shock wave therapy 136
shower (penis size) 35, 44
Siffredi, Rocco 57
sildenafil citrate *see* Viagra
silicone
extender 177–178
implant 132
injections 65
prosthesis 70, *71*
ring 154–155
size of penis 15, 35, 38–60; *see also* erection; megaphallus; microphallus
aging 191
apparent length 50
average 42, 44–49, 63
at birth 52
blood type, effects 42
body size, in relation to 43
body weight and 50–51
dietary supplements 63–64
endocrine disruptors 58, 60
and ethnicity 51–52
extenders 67–68
gel to enlarge 64
increasing 61–75
injections to enlarge 65–66
jelqing to enlarge 75
liposuction 69–70, 71
Manning Index 59–60
measurement 39–43, 41, 45
penile dysmorphic disorder 63
penoplasty 70–74

puberty 58
pumps to enlarge 68
snake bite to enlarge 66
studies 40–44
surgery 69–74
visible length 50
weights to enlarge 66–67
skin grafts 164–165
Skoptsy sect 147
slang for penis 200–202
smegma 16, 77, 159, 186–188
snails 26
snake 30
bite 66
soft enhancement of
   percutaneous absorption
   (SEPA) 135
Spanish fly 122
sperm 14, 24, 32, 37, 58,
   145–146, 171; *see also*
   ejaculation
spicule 29
spider bite and erectile
   dysfunction 137–138
splitting, penis 140
sports, 176 178
spotted hyena 27
stem cells 65, 163
Stendra 125
Stigler 51
strangulation, penile 154–155
stress, effect on penis 15,
   39, 41
subincision 152, *153*
sunburn 84–85
surgery *see also* circumcision
to enlarge penis 69–74
sex reassignment 147
transplant, penile 167–173
suspensory ligament 14, *15*,
   70, *71*
synthetic foreskin 166
syphilis 81–83

T
tadalafil 125
taghaandan 88
tanning the penis 20–21,
   84–85
tattoos 153–154
testicles 86, 117, 147, 171,
   173
testicular cancer 58
testosterone 20, 53, 62, 191

ADAM 193, 195–199
theft of penises 111–112
thickness of penis *see* size of
   penis
tobacco use and erectile
   dysfunction 119, 136
Topiglan 136
Toulouse-Lautrec, Henri de
   54–55
transplant, penile 167–173
Treponema pallidum 82
trinitrin 134–135
Tucano people (Colombia) 38
tunica albuginea *13*, 14, 74,
   87, 89, 96, 192
Tupinambá people (Brazil)
   66
TUX (tuxedo for penis) 180

U
ultrasound 21, 88, 136
ultraviolet rays 20–21
urethra *13*, 14, *15*, 16, *19*,
   92, 93, 99, 103, 108–111,
   147, 151
epispadias 86–87
erection 32
fractures 87–89
hypospadias 91–93
jewelry 141
MUSE 131–132
penile strangulation 154–155
plugs 141
subincision 152–153
urethritis 78, 108–111
urinary meatus 17, *17*, 135,
   146, 152

V
vacuums 126; *see* pumps
vardenafil 125
Veale, David 43
veins
circumflex 32, 33
dorsal 13, *13*, 19, 32
Viagra 34–35, 93, 104,
   123–125
Viagra condoms 134–135
Vitaros 135
vitiligo 20

W
Wake Forest Institute for
   Regenerative Medicine

(WFIRM) 172
wandering spider 137–138
warts, genital 83–84
water bugs 29
weight, body 50–51, 69–70
weights to elongate penis 56,
   66–67
whale, blue 23–24
Willy Warmer 181

X
X-ray of penis 21
xenotransplantation, penile
   168, 173

Z
Zanifil 134–135